Obesity in the Black Community

This landmark textbook, written by three leading experts in obesity medicine, provides a comprehensive examination of the complexities, challenges, and opportunities in addressing obesity within Black communities. By exploring the interplay of biopsychosocial factors and cultural dynamics, this authoritative resource presents a forward-thinking, evidence-led approach to one of the most critical public health issues of our time.

Grounded in the latest research and enriched by clinical expertise, the book offers actionable strategies for healthcare professionals seeking to deliver culturally sensitive and effective care. With a focus on addressing health disparities and dismantling harmful stereotypes, this text sets a new benchmark for equitable and impactful obesity treatment.

Key Features

- Challenges misconceptions and biases to offer practical, solutions-driven approaches to obesity care
- Combines clinical best practices with cultural competence to enhance patient engagement and outcomes
- Features contributions from Black physicians, providing valuable insights that blend lived experience with professional expertise

Ideal for medical students, clinicians, and healthcare professionals, this essential guide is also a vital resource for researchers and public health advocates dedicated to advancing health equity and improving outcomes for historically underserved populations.

Obesity in the Black Community

Weighing the Complexity above Statistics

Kathi Earles

MD, MPH, DABOM

Tiffani Bell-Washington

MD, MPH, MBA, FAPA, FOMA, DABOM, DABLM

Sylvia Gonsahn-Bollie

MD, DABOM, FOMA

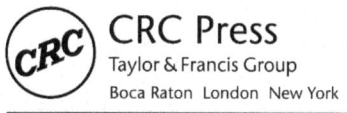

CRC Press
Taylor & Francis Group
Boca Raton London New York

CRC Press is an imprint of the
Taylor & Francis Group, an **informa** business

Designed cover image: Jordan Ross

First edition published 2026
by CRC Press
2385 NW Executive Center Drive, Suite 320, Boca Raton, FL 33431

and by CRC Press
4 Park Square, Milton Park, Abingdon, Oxon, OX14 4RN

CRC Press is an imprint of Taylor & Francis Group, LLC

© 2026 Kathi Earles, Tiffani Bell-Washington, and Sylvia Gonsahn-Bollie

ISBN: 978-1-032-62196-8 (hbk)
ISBN: 978-1-032-62194-4 (pbk)
ISBN: 978-1-032-62221-7 (ebk)

DOI: 10.1201/9781032622217

Typeset in Sabon
by Apex CoVantage, LLC

My deepest gratitude goes to:

God for making all of this and much more possible. Mom and Dad for your unwavering love and support on earth and in heaven. My Allie for lovingly, patiently, and graciously sharing your life with me. Jordan, Riley, and Jax for the sensational joy and honor of being your Mom. And to my Sorors, my ride or die HU Bison crew, my Zion Hill family, my chosen sisters and brothers, and all who graciously shared space with me, my light is brighter because you shared yours with me.

Kathi Earles, MD, MPH, DABOM

My deepest gratitude goes to:

My mom, for your sacrifices, pursuit of excellence, and insistence that I do the same. My sister, for being my example of Black Excellence and paving the way. My family members, especially my dad, whose loss to obesity and preventable chronic diseases fuels my passion for increasing health and longevity in our community. Greg, Isaiah, Naomi, Imani, Natali, and Bethani, for your endless love, adventures, and being my unwavering source of joy and inspiration. My patients, mentors, colleagues, sister friends, and Sorors, for teaching me the power of unity and shared purpose. God, thank you for being my strength and shield, and for showing me that through faith, all things are possible.

Tiffani Bell-Washington, MD, MPH, MBA, FAPA, FOMA, DABOM, DABLM

My deepest gratitude goes to:

My Grandma Sylvia for teaching me to see beyond the physical. My parents and sister for never giving up on me. Rodney Bollie for your love and support. "Zee" and "Kehzie" for your patience and encouragement. My dear sister friends and every patient who's trusted me with their care. God thank you for making "All things possible" in my life through Christ.

Sylvia Gonsahn-Bollie, MD, DABOM, FOMA

Contents

TIFFANI BELL-WASHINGTON, MD, MPH, MBA, FAPA, FOMA, DABOM, DABLM,
JOYNITA R. NICHOLSON, DO, DABOM, FOMA, AND
SYLVIA GONSAHN-BOLLIE, MD, DABOM, FOMA

KATHI EARLES, MD, MPH, DABOM AND
SYLVIA GONSAHN-BOLLIE, MD, DABOM, FOMA

8 Nutrition and Lifestyle Intervention and Inclusive Obesity Care

62

DAPHNE BRYAN, MD, DABOM,

TIFFANI BELL-WASHINGTON MD, MPH, MBA, FAPA, FOMA, DABOM, DABLM, AND

SYLVIA GONSAHN-BOLLIE, MD, DABOM, FOMA

9 Behavioral Impact and Interventions in the Treatment of Obesity

72

TIFFANI BELL-WASHINGTON, MD, MPH, MBA, FAPA, FOMA, DABOM, DABLM,

SYLVIA GONSAHN-BOLLIE, MD, DABOM, FOMA, AND

SHARON DODD, MD

Foreword

Fatima Cody Stanford
MD, MPH, MPA, MBA, MACP, FAAP, FAHA, FAMWA, FTOS

Obesity is a complex and chronic disease that permeates every facet of a person's health and well-being. It is a condition that disproportionately impacts the Black community, a reality exacerbated by persistent stigma, misconceptions, and systemic inequities. As a physician–scientist specializing in obesity medicine, I am acutely aware of the imperative to approach this disease with scientific rigor and cultural humility. The authors of this book have embarked on an inspiring journey to provide essential education, hope, and solutions for healthcare clinicians dedicated to making a meaningful difference in the lives of Black patients.

This book addresses a critical gap in medical literature. Obesity treatment is not a one-size-fits-all approach. Yet, for many years, research and clinical guidelines have largely overlooked the unique social, cultural, and environmental factors that shape health outcomes in the Black community. The authors understand this reality deeply. With their expertise, passion, and dedication, they have created a guide that offers clinical insights and acknowledges and respects the lived experiences of Black patients grappling with obesity.

As you delve into this book, you will discover evidence-based strategies tailored to resonate with Black families and communities. More importantly, you will witness the authors' unwavering commitment to addressing the complex web of factors contributing to obesity in this population—whether it's socioeconomic barriers, cultural dietary norms, or the historical and ongoing impact of racism and bias in healthcare. Their passion for improving the health and well-being of Black people is palpable on every page, and their goal is clear: to provide tools that empower healthcare professionals to help their patients reclaim their health and live their fullest, healthiest lives.

Obesity is a disease, not a character flaw. It is a condition that warrants treatment with the same urgency, respect, and evidence-based care as any other chronic illness. Yet, for too many in the Black community, this reality is obscured by stigma and misunderstanding. The authors' tireless efforts to dismantle these barriers are not only commendable—they are essential. This book is a testament to their courage, their expertise, and their belief that by transforming the way we approach obesity treatment, we can transform lives.

I am honored to support this work and to witness the change it will inspire. For every clinician who reads these pages, may it strengthen your resolve to see and treat your patients with the empathy, respect, and dignity they deserve. And for every patient whose story and struggle are reflected here, may this book serve as a reminder that you are not alone, your health matters, and a community of advocates is fighting for you every step of the way.

Together, we can change the narrative of obesity in the Black community and, in doing so, bring health and hope to those who need it most.

Preface

We are at a pivotal moment in history for both the Black community and healthcare. The COVID-19 pandemic exposed and amplified long-standing health disparities, leading to disproportionately higher death rates in the Black community. Over the past five years, we have endured a global pandemic, witnessed senseless killings that ignited the rallying cry of "Black Lives Matter," and seen a resurgence of overt racism. Yet, alongside these challenges, we have also celebrated moments of resilience and progress—Justice Ketanji Brown Jackson became the first Black woman appointed to the U.S. Supreme Court, Kamala Harris became the first Black U.S. Vice President, and 15-year-old Heman Bekele was named *Time* magazine's Kid of the Year for inventing a cancer-curing soap. These triumphs reflect the richness of Black culture and the strength of the Black community, especially in times of crisis.

As we emerge from the trials of the past few years, we face a new health crisis: obesity. Now, more than ever, we need the collective strength of our community to meet this challenge head-on. As Black women and obesity specialists, we have witnessed the profound impact of obesity on individuals and families—both in our personal lives and in clinical practice.

Despite having the highest rates of obesity in the United States, the Black community lacks a comprehensive, evidence-based resource that explores how this disease uniquely affects us. Writing this book was both a daunting and necessary task. We acknowledge that no single book can capture the full diversity of the Black experience, and we do not pretend that this work is complete. To truly reflect the Black community would require volumes. We also hope that one day, this book will become obsolete, as healthcare advances beyond the need to define care by race.

Fortunately, science now confirms what many of us have long known: obesity is not a lifestyle choice, but a complex, multifactorial disease. Within the Black community, the challenges associated with obesity are compounded by historical, social, and cultural factors.

As we developed this book, we drew from our professional expertise, the latest research, the support of our colleagues, and most importantly, our personal experiences with obesity. We write not just as clinicians and obesity experts, but as daughters, mothers, sisters, and wives, who have each personally lost a loved one due to complications of obesity and health disparities. Despite the adversity of the past, we remain confident that the Black community can rise above stagnant statistics. Together, we can embrace innovative solutions and overcome obesity to achieve optimal health and wellness. We believe in the strength of the Black community and are hopeful for a healthier future.

Authors

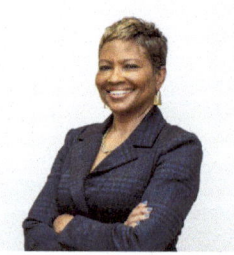

Dr. Kathi Earles MD, MPH, DABOM is the Executive Obesity Medical Liaison for the South Coast region of Novo Nordisk, Inc. Prior to the this role, she was the Assistant Director of the Morehouse School of Medicine (MSM) Pediatrics Residency program, where she was instrumental in developing the curriculum and establishing the program from its inception. She continues to be an active faculty member at MSM, where she participates in residency and graduate medical education and serves as an adjunct faculty member in the Department of Pediatrics. Dr. Earles graduated from Howard University, where she received a Bachelor of Science in Microbiology with a minor in Chemistry. After graduating from Howard University College of Medicine in 1991, she pursued a residency program at the University of Southern California in Los Angeles, California. She later received a Masters in Public Health from the University of California Los Angeles, after which she assumed the position of Assistant Residency Program Director at Morehouse School of Medicine. She is a highly respected speaker, writer, and educator on pediatric obesity and has a particular interest in the health disparities impacting minority communities. She has authored several publications, including a chapter entitled "Epidemic on Overweight and Obesity" in *Health Disparities* with Dr. David Satcher, former Surgeon General. Dr. Earles is also published in the field of pediatric obesity, including *Scale Back! Why Childhood Obesity Is Not Just about Weight*, which she co-authored with Dr. Sandra Moore. The book is designed to address the epidemic of pediatric obesity and identify solutions suited for the lay community.

Dr. Earles enjoys reading, exercising, traveling, art, and cheering for the Atlanta Dream. She and her husband currently reside in Atlanta, Georgia.

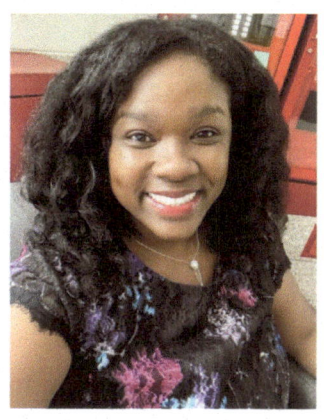

Dr. Tiffani Bell-Washington MD, MPH, MBA, FAPA, FOMA, DABOM, DABLM is a Harvard-trained public health expert and quadruple board-certified physician in Psychiatry, Child & Adolescent Psychiatry, Obesity Medicine, and Lifestyle Medicine. She is the founder of The Healthy Weigh MD, a concierge mental health and weight management practice delivering culturally responsive, stigma-free care for women and children.

A nationally recognized speaker on the intersection of obesity and mental health, Dr. Bell-Washington is widely known for her advocacy to dismantle weight stigma and expand access to equitable, evidence-informed care. She has been featured by both Harvard and Yale for her work advancing health equity and training clinician-entrepreneurs. She has created content on the intersection of obesity and mental health for the Obesity Society, Obesity Medicine Association, and local outlets. Dr. Bell-Washington is also the founder of the Bell Well Joy Initiative, a platform dedicated to spreading joy, reducing burnout, and helping professionals reclaim purpose and balance. With an Executive MBA from Yale, she empowers physicians to build joyful, mission-driven businesses rooted in integrity and well-being.

Her award-winning leadership has earned numerous honors, including the National Medical Association's "Top Physician under 40," the National Minority Quality Forum's 40 Under 40 in Minority Health, and the 2025 Early Career Physician of the Year Award from the American Medical Women's Association..

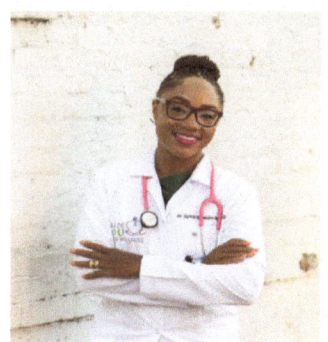

Dr. Sylvia Gonsahn-Bollie MD, DABOM, FOMA is a dual board-certified obesity and internal medicine physician, clinical researcher, bestselling author, and nationally recognized advocate for health equity. Her work has been featured in Forbes, the *Wall Street Journal*, and other major outlets. She is the founder of Embrace You Weight & Wellness, an initiative focused on culturally tailored obesity education and whole-person care.

Dr. Gonsahn-Bollie authored *Embrace You: Your Guide to Transforming Weight Loss Misconceptions into Lifelong Wellness*, named one of Healthline's "Best Weight Loss Books of 2022" and Livestrong's "Top 8 Weight Loss Books of 2022." She has developed content for Black Health, BlackDoctor.org, and served as a local leader with the Black Physicians Healthcare Network and Walk With a Doc. She previously served on the Board of Trustees for the Obesity Medicine Association, helping shape the direction of obesity care.

Currently, Dr. Gonsahn-Bollie is a full-time clinical researcher in obesity drug development and continues her community health equity efforts by leading a Walk With a Doc group in Montgomery County, MD, as well as speaking and writing to empower individuals through personalized, culturally tailored obesity education.

Introduction

Sunday Dinner

Reverend Williams sits down at the family table, his plate piled high with steaming collard greens cooked with fatback, mashed potatoes swimming in gravy, and a mountain of cornbread. He surveys the feast before him, satisfied with the abundance. Before he begins, he closes his eyes and offers a lighthearted prayer to the Divine: "Bless this bread, bless this meat, bless this belly, 'cause I's gon' eat!" With the prayer said, he digs in, savoring each bite.

This scene from the movie *Soul Food* (Tilman & Tillman, 1997) captures the deep connection between Black families, cultural traditions, and food. The film highlights both the joy and complexity of Black family gatherings, with food at the center of celebration, connection, and legacy. Yet amid the laughter and family drama, the movie touches on a sobering reality. The beloved family matriarch, Big Mama, dies from complications of type 2 diabetes—her life marked by a long history of obesity and its associated conditions.

Big Mama's passing is a tragedy that leaves a void her family struggles to fill. Her character reflects the experiences of many Black Americans navigating obesity and chronic illnesses, including type 2 diabetes, cardiovascular disease, sleep apnea, and depression. As healthcare clinicians, many of us will encounter individuals like Big Mama or Reverend Williams, either during the early stages of obesity or while treating the comorbidities that often follow. These encounters challenge us to adopt a compassionate, culturally sensitive, and evidence-based approach to care.

A Vision for Culturally Responsive Care

In clinical settings, healing begins the moment a patient enters a welcoming environment. From inclusive seating that accommodates all body types to culturally relevant artwork, every detail signals respect and belonging. When greeted warmly by staff and handed a gown that fits comfortably, patients experience dignity and ease. The care journey continues with a clinician who listens attentively, acknowledges the patient's concerns without judgment, and engages in a collaborative conversation about health and wellness.

In this context, obesity care goes beyond simply addressing weight. Clinicians deconstruct the disease of obesity, explaining the complex interplay of genetic, environmental, and behavioral factors that influence health outcomes. Through shared dialogue, patients are empowered to understand their condition, reducing the stigma and biases often associated with obesity. Treatment plans are developed together, incorporating behavioral therapy, culturally sensitive dietary recommendations, exercise plans tailored to individual abilities, and referrals to dietitians, physical therapists, or mental health professionals when needed.

When appropriate, clinicians discuss anti-obesity medications or surgical options aligned with the patient's health goals and preferences. Frequent follow-ups foster encouragement, accountability, and a sense of partnership, ensuring long-term success. This holistic, culturally responsive approach not only improves individual outcomes but also strengthens the health of families and communities.

Reimagining Traditions for a Healthier Future

What if the next chapter of *Soul Food* told a different story? Imagine Reverend Williams and his family gathered around the same table, but with a new twist on their cherished traditions. Instead of fatback, smoked turkey flavors the collard greens. Whole grain or sweet potato muffins replace cornbread, and mashed cauliflower stands in for mashed potatoes. After a shared prayer, the family enjoys these new dishes in appropriate portions, balancing tradition with health-conscious choices. Laughter fills the room as they tell stories of Big Mama, honoring her memory with gratitude for the healthier future they are building together.

A Call to Action

This book, *Obesity in the Black Community*, provides healthcare clinicians and community advocates with the tools to create that future. Through a comprehensive exploration of the origins, obstacles, and opportunities surrounding obesity in the Black community, this book offers practical strategies for delivering culturally tailored care. The clinical considerations checklists in each chapter are designed to be quick references that help facilitate conversations rooted in empathy and cultural understanding.

Our hope is that this book will empower clinicians to make meaningful connections with patients, reduce health disparities, and improve the lives of individuals and families alike. By embracing culturally relevant care, we can change the narrative of obesity—transforming it from one of tragedy and loss into one of healing, empowerment, and joy.

Together, we can build healthier communities, one patient, one family, and one office visit at a time.

Section 1

Origins

Chapter 1

Who Is Black?

*Sylvia Gonsahn-Bollie, MD, DABOM, FOMA and
Kathi Earles, MD, MPH, DABOM*

> It is racism, not "race," that causes differences in health outcomes between racial groups.
>
> —Yin Paradies, 2015

Chapter 1 Highlights

- **Race is a social construct** that influences disproportionate obesity care in the self-identified or labeled Black community.
- The evidence is clear: **Black/African American people are not biologically disadvantaged.** Rather, the impact of racism and its extensive effects exacerbates any individual risk associated with excess adiposity and obesity.
- **As medicine evolves past race-based care,** the influence of race and racism in obesity care requires that clinicians are aware of their implicit bias as well as explicit weight bias and engage in shared decision-making with patients.

INTRODUCTION

The discussion of race is inseparable from racism. So, to discuss obesity in the Black community, we must start by acknowledging the significant impact racism has had on the obesity epidemic. Scholars in other disciplines have used the influence of racism on the obesity epidemic to refute the health impact of obesity on Black people (Strings, 2020). However, given the evidence of the increased all-cause mortality associated with obesity—especially at a BMI greater than 35—medically, it would be a disservice not to address the impact of obesity on Blacks (Byrd et al., 2018). However, any discussions of obesity in the Black community must occur from a comprehensive, biopsychosocial perspective that starts with acknowledging the origin of race

DOI: 10.1201/9781032622217-2

and the limitations of its use in healthcare when diagnosing and treating obesity. This chapter will discuss the following:

- The Intersection of Obesity, Race, and Social Constructs
- Race and Racism in Obesity Medicine
- Evolving beyond Race-Based Healthcare in Obesity Treatment
- Clinical Considerations Checklist: Discussing Race in Obesity Care

THE INTERSECTION OF OBESITY, RACE, AND SOCIAL CONSTRUCTS

In 2013, the American Medical Association officially recognized obesity as "a disease state with multiple pathophysiological aspects requiring a range of interventions to advance obesity treatment and prevention" (American Medical Association, 2019). However, it's essential to recognize that the treatment of obesity has been influenced by historical misconceptions surrounding race. Race is a social construct, not a biological reality, despite centuries of misinformation about its biological basis (NIH, Human Genome Project). Therefore, "race is a social construct" has become a common academic and intellectual catchphrase. Yet due to generations of racial misinformation and implicit bias, many clinicians and patients may struggle to understand the concept in clinical practice (Hall et al., 2015).

Here is an illustrative example from a news story: Several years ago, a prominent chapter of a historically African American organization was led by a dynamic woman with almond skin complexion and brown curly hair. When it was revealed the organization's president had been born White or Caucasian, the organization and the public were shocked. She had made physical changes (curly extensions and skin bronzer) to appear Black or African American. By assuming a Black racial identity, she improved her social status within a prestigious historical organization. Perhaps this story was shocking because it was a case of a White person assuming a Black racial identity for social gain. However, the reverse, the necessity of a Black person assuming a White racial identity, or "passing," has been a widely understood practice in the Black community, especially during slavery and Jim Crow. The concept of racial categorization based on skin color was invented for socio-political power. Race and biological misinformation were used as justification for European colonialism, the trans-Atlantic slave trade, White supremacy, segregation, and more. Unlike race, ethnicity is defined as cultural factors such as ancestry, cuisine, nationality, language, and/or religion (Lewis et al., 2023), shared by specific communities. Ethnicity will be discussed in more detail in Chapter 2, "What Is the Black Community?"

RACE AND RACISM IN OBESITY MEDICINE: HISTORICAL AND CONTEMPORARY PERSPECTIVES

In medicine, race was used as justification for dehumanization. Black people were subjected to unethical medical experiments during slavery and beyond. Most notorious was the U.S. Public Health Service's Untreated Syphilis Study at the Tuskegee Institute, in which lifesaving syphilis treatment was withheld from Black patients to observe the natural course of the disease (CDC, 2022). Throughout history, racism in science and medicine established a pattern where Black people were used for disease experimentation but excluded from measures to prevent or treat disease.

For the disease of obesity, Black people were not included in the population used to create the standard body mass index (BMI) table of the "normal weight range" (Strings, 2019a). Later chapters will explore the flaws of BMI, especially for individual use, since it is a population-based tool. However, it is essential to note the absence of Black people and other diverse groups from the BMI dataset. Diversity must be considered when using BMI as a screening tool, especially in the Black community. Researchers such as Dr. Fatima Cody Stanford have proposed updated BMI charts adjusted for race, ethnicity, and obesity-related conditions (Stanford et al., 2019). Additionally, more accurate measurements of adiposity, such as waist circumference and body composition, are critical for individualized care. However, even these metrics lack sufficient validation for Black populations (Katzmarzyk et al., 2018). One example is the adjusted measurements based on geographical location and ethnicity waist circumference proposed by the International Diabetes Federation. Currently, the sub-Saharan African population is "awaiting more specific data."

New research from the Pennington Center Longitudinal Study suggests that sub-Saharan African women may not develop insulin resistance until their waist circumference reaches 38 inches, compared to the standard threshold of 35 inches (Kabakambira et al., 2018). This finding highlights the limitations of current obesity standards, which may not adequately reflect the health risks of diverse populations. It underscores the need for population-specific measures rather than assumptions based on race alone. Obesity is a complex disease requiring multiple biological, psychological, and environmental factors.

Although biological and psychological factors play significant roles in obesity development, research shows that an obesogenic environment is more likely to increase obesity rates. Due to systemic racism, African Americans are more likely to live in obesogenic environments with higher barriers to health, such as food deserts, unsafe neighborhoods, and financial insecurity. These disparities are the result of race-driven policies such as redlining and rezoning, which have exacerbated the social determinants of health (SDOH) in Black communities (Bell et al., 2019). Chapter 4, "The Role of Social

Determinants of Health on the Disease of Obesity," will explore these issues in further detail.

A consensus statement released in 2022 by six leading U.S.-based organizations reflects the shift toward more equitable obesity care:

> Obesity is a highly prevalent chronic disease characterized by excessive fat accumulation or distribution that presents a risk to health and requires lifelong care. Virtually every system in the body is affected by obesity. Major chronic diseases associated with obesity include diabetes, heart disease, and cancer. The body mass index (weight in kg/height in meters^2) is used to screen for obesity, but it does not displace clinical judgment. BMI is not a measure of body fat. Social determinants, race, ethnicity, and age may modify the risk associated with a given BMI. Bias and stigmatization directed at people with obesity contribute to poor health and impair treatment. Every person with obesity should have access to evidence-based treatment.
>
> (Obesity Medicine Association, 2022)

This statement marks a step toward addressing the bias of the past and recognizing the importance of personalized, culturally competent care. However, more work is needed to dismantle the systemic barriers that continue to shape health outcomes for Black individuals with obesity.

EVOLVING BEYOND RACE-BASED HEALTHCARE IN OBESITY TREATMENT

Returning to the story of the White woman who "passed" for Black. Although she may have done so for short-term political gain, the case could also be used to highlight race as a social construct and the health inequity that exists for the Black community. This news story was juicy gossip for talk shows, but from a medical perspective, the health implications of this deception were concerning. By labeling herself as a Black woman, she had already significantly worsened her health, not by changing her biology but by simply calling herself Black. Specifically, if she had obesity, by calling herself a Black woman she had increased her 3.05% chances of dying from obesity complications as a White woman to 18% as a Black woman (Okobi et al., 2023). This is the flaw in race-based healthcare: Her biology did not change, but her health risks did all because of her perceived skin color. According to the Human Genome Project, "There is more genetic variation within self-identified racial groups than between them. . . . There is 99.9% shared biological identity amongst all humans" (Taylor et al., 2024). It is important to note that differences in the expression level of certain genes associated with appetite regulation and obesity, such as BNDF and SEMA4D, have been seen in Blacks and African Americans (Byrd et al.,

2018). However, different expression levels of the same genes are also seen in people with a higher BMI or obesity. Chapter 3, "Obesity as a Disease," will discuss this topic in greater detail. It is essential to consider all the factors that can contribute to higher rates of obesity in the Black community and individuals instead of simply searching for race-based biological findings.

The evidence is clear: Black/African American people are not biologically disadvantaged. Rather, the impact of racism and its extensive effects exacerbates any individual risk associated with excess adiposity and obesity (Byrd et al., 2018). Medicine and healthcare must acknowledge the harmful influence of racism on obesity. The data is clear: It is time to evolve beyond using race as a health indicator. Research must focus on developing comprehensive assessments beyond the color of one's skin. The incorporation of mixed-variable scoring systems that include geographic factors and other social determinants of health is promising. However, at the time of this publication, such tools are not used in daily clinical use. Currently, science and healthcare exist in tension between the biased data of the past, harmful health inequity, and self-identified Black people who want and deserve better health. There is still widespread racial, gender, and weight bias that impacts Black people with obesity disproportionately.

CONCLUSION

For now, there are signs that obesity medicine is starting to reckon with the biases of the past. In 2022, six leading U.S.-based organizations released a consensus statement on obesity that highlights the complexity of the disease of obesity, limitations of the body mass index, and the impact of bias on people with obesity and from different ethnicities. This evolving perspective offers hope for a future where comprehensive, culturally tailored, and individualized obesity care becomes the norm.

While there is a need for systematic changes at every level of society to fully address the effects of racism on disparities in obesity rates and treatment in Black people, in this book we start with the doctor–patient, or more broadly, clinician–patient, relationship.

For clinicians, change starts with:

1. Acknowledging how historical biases impact Black healthcare, especially in obesity treatment.
2. Accessing personal implicit bias through the Harvard Implicit Association Test.
3. Increasing their knowledge base to address misinformation.
4. Asking permission and having an open dialogue with patients about the impact of race on their health and how it may be incorporated into their care.

The Clinical Considerations Checklist included in this chapter offers a starting point for these discussions. However, we anticipate that emerging scientific and technological advances will soon allow healthcare to move beyond race and other socially constructed characteristics altogether.

The journey toward equitable healthcare is ongoing, and addressing the systemic barriers that Black individuals face will require sustained efforts. With a focus on clinician–patient relationships, we can begin to close the gaps and provide the personalized care that every patient deserves.

CLINICAL CONSIDERATIONS CHECKLIST: DISCUSSING RACE IN OBESITY CARE

Chapter 1 of *Origins, Obstacles, and Opportunities: Clinical Guide to Obesity and the Black Community* discussed the origins and impact of race and racism on obesity in the Black community. Race-based medical care is harmful and leads to worse health outcomes. Effective obesity care must address the health disparities caused by racism and evolve to personalized care. Healthcare professionals may not be familiar with how to have conversations with patients on race, racism, and the impact on obesity care.

This checklist is intended for clinicians and patients to use together to discuss the patient's personalized perception and key considerations in the incorporation of race, ethnicity, and culture in obesity care.

Key Clinical Facts on Obesity and Race as of 2024

Body Mass Index (BMI) is the most common screening tool for obesity. However, the standard BMI chart may be inaccurate for most Black people. Culturally tailored BMI charts have been proposed.

	BMI (kg/m²)					
	Men			Women		
Obesity Comorbidity	Black	Hispanic	White	Black	Hispanic	White
Hypertension	28	29	28	31	28	27
Dyslipidemia	27	26	27	29	27	25
Diabetes	29	29	30	33	30	29
≥2 risk factors	28	29	29	31	30	28
Average	28	28	29	31	29	27

Abbreviation: BMI, Body Mass Index.
Source: Stanford et al. (2019). "Race, Ethnicity, Sex, and Obesity: Is It Time to Personalize the Scale?" Mayo Clin Proc. 94(2):362–369.

Evolving Medical Care from Race-Based to Personalized Care

- *Individualized measures of excess adiposity (extra fat)*: Body Composition (Body Fat %; Lean Mass); Waist Circumference; Cardiovascular Health; Metabolic Health
- *Individualized care must incorporate all aspects of health*: Physical, mental, and spiritual, as well as public health considerations such as where one is born, lives, works, plays, and worships ("Social Determinants of Health")

Clinical Discussion Points

Do you self-identify with a specific racial/ethnic group? If so, what group:

_____

How important is it to you that I incorporate your racial or ethnic identity into your care?

0 1 2 3 4 5 6 7 8 9 10
Not   Very
at all   Important

Have you or has anyone close to you ever had a negative healthcare experience due to race?

_____

_____

_____

What can your doctor/clinician do to help you feel seen and heard during your healthcare journey?

_____

_____

_____

Patient Resource

Obesity Action Coalition. (2021). Obesity and weight bias in racial and ethnic groups. Retrieved from https://www.obesityaction.org/resources/obesity-and-weight-bias-in-racial-and-ethnic-groups/

Clinician Resource

U.S. Department of Health and Human Services. (n.d.). Think Cultural Health. Retrieved from https://cccm.thinkculturalhealth.hhs.gov/

Chapter 2

What Is the Black Community?

Sylvia Gonsahn-Bollie, MD, DABOM, FOMA,
Kathi Earles, MD, MPH, DABOM, and
Tiffani Bell-Washington, MD, MPH, MBA, FAPA,
FOMA, DABOM, DABLM

> The Black community is not a monolith; it is a mosaic of lived experiences, histories, and cultures.
>
> —Unknown

Chapter 2 Highlights

- **The Black Community is Diverse:** There is no single definition of the Black community; it is shaped by cultural heritage, geography, and shared experiences.
- **Community vs. Culture:** Understanding the distinction between community (shared space and goals) and culture (traditions and practices) is key for effective engagement.
- **Historical and Sociological Origins Matter:** The legacies of slavery, segregation, and systemic racism continue to influence the structure of Black communities and their healthcare needs.

INTRODUCTION

If you ask a group of people, "What is the Black community?" each individual's response would vary widely. The answers may depend on many factors, such as the individual's cultural background, geographic location, age, life experiences, and more. This diversity of responses is a testament to the complexity and richness of the Black community, which defies a single definition.

For healthcare professionals, this variability is a critical insight. Too often, clinicians approach the "Black community" as a monolithic entity, which can lead to unconscious bias, perpetuating stereotypes, and misinformed care decisions. The reality is that the Black community is heterogenous—shaped by historical events, sociological factors, geographic diversity, and a broad range of cultural influences. Understanding this complexity is vital to providing equitable and culturally responsive care.

DOI: 10.1201/9781032622217-3

HISTORICAL ORIGINS: THE AFRICAN DIASPORA

The foundation of what we now call the Black community lies in the African Diaspora—a term that captures the forced migration of Africans across the world through slavery and colonization. However, the Diaspora also represents the resilience and adaptability of African cultures as they were transplanted into new lands, often under brutal conditions. In new geographic locations, African culture melded with the local customs and cultures to create a distinct Black community in that region. Today's diversity within the Black community can be traced back to this multifaceted history (Rotimi et al., 2016).

Over generations, the descendants of enslaved Africans in the United States developed their own identities, traditions, and cultural practices. These expressions are both a response to systemic oppression and a celebration of survival and resistance. Yet, the origins of the trans-Atlantic slave trade forcibly transplanting millions of Africans to America under horrific conditions lays the groundwork for the multifactorial disparities (health, socioeconomic) that persist today (Yancy, 2020). Understanding the African Diaspora's role is essential for any clinician seeking to grasp the historical roots of the Black community. For a more in-depth understanding of this topic, read *The African Diaspora: History, Adaptation, and Health* by Rotimi et al. (2016).

The Great Migration—one of the largest demographic shifts in U.S. history—saw millions of African Americans move from the rural South to urban centers in the North and West. This migration reshaped the demographics and social structures of cities such as Chicago, Detroit, and Los Angeles and led to the formation of vibrant Black communities in these cities and others. These urban enclaves became cultural and political hubs, fostering a distinct Black identity. However, even in these new environments, Black communities faced redlining and exclusion from economic opportunities, leading to concentrated increased rates of overcrowding, poverty, and health disparities that persist today (Chatters et al., 2021).

SOCIOLOGICAL ORIGINS: FROM SLAVERY TO REDLINING

Sociologically, the development of the Black community has been deeply influenced by systemic racism. The legacies of slavery, segregation, and discriminatory practices like redlining have all left enduring marks on the social and economic status of Black people in America and throughout the Diaspora.

These sociological factors are not just historical footnotes; they actively shape the health outcomes, healthcare access, and overall well-being of the Black community today.

COMMUNITY VS. CULTURE: WHAT'S THE DIFFERENCE?

Understanding the difference between "community" and "culture" is key:

- *Community* refers to a group of people with shared experiences, values, and goals. It's often rooted in shared geography, social networks, or institutional affiliations. A person's community is where they find belonging and support.
- *Culture*, on the other hand, is the set of beliefs, practices, customs, and traditions that are passed down within a group. Culture can transcend geography and is often tied to historical and ancestral roots. For example, African American culture includes shared artistic expressions such as jazz, hip-hop, and spoken word poetry.

Although community and culture overlap, they are not synonymous. One person can belong to multiple communities while sharing a broader cultural heritage. For example, a Black physician might belong to both a professional community (like a Black medical association) and a religious community, while also identifying with broader African American culture (Lofton et al., 2023).

A key concept in understanding the Black community is "social capital"—the networks, relationships, and norms that enable cooperation and support within a community. In Black communities, social capital has been a vital resource for coping with adversity and promoting health. Black churches and community organizations often play central roles in providing social support, health education, and advocacy. However, the erosion of social capital due to economic decline and urbanization has weakened the fabric of some Black communities, making it more challenging to address health disparities, including obesity (Curry and Larkin, 2002).

EXAMPLES OF DIVERSE BLACK COMMUNITIES

The term "Black community" is often used as a catch-all phrase, but it encompasses a wide variety of groups with distinct identities. Here are a few examples:

1. *African American Communities*: Descendants of enslaved Africans brought to the United States. Cultural traditions are rooted in the unique history of Black Americans, with influences ranging from gospel music to soul food.
2. *Afro-Caribbean Communities*: Comprising immigrants from countries such as Jamaica, Haiti, and Trinidad, these communities bring diverse languages, religious practices, and cultural norms.

3. *African Immigrant Communities*: More recent immigrants from countries such as Nigeria, Ghana, Ethiopia, and Somalia have formed vibrant communities with their own distinct cultural practices, languages, and community structures.
4. *Afro-Latinx Communities*: People of African descent from Latin America, such as those from Brazil, Colombia, or the Dominican Republic, often maintain a blended identity that incorporates both Latin and African traditions.

The way individuals decide which community they belong to is often shaped by several factors: cultural heritage, shared experiences, language, religion, and sometimes even geography. For example, a Nigerian immigrant might feel a stronger sense of belonging to other Nigerians in their local area rather than to the broader African American community, due to shared language and cultural traditions.

IMPACT OF COMMUNITY ON HEALTHCARE

The Black community significantly influences healthcare, particularly in how cultural norms, beliefs, and practices shape health behaviors and access to care. To provide effective healthcare to Black patients, it is essential to understand and respect these norms.

For example, traditional dietary practices within the Black community often include foods that are high in fat and sugar, contributing to the prevalence of obesity and related health conditions such as diabetes and hypertension. Addressing these health issues requires culturally tailored interventions that recognize the cultural significance of these foods while promoting healthier alternatives (Thorpe et al., 2021).

Trust in the healthcare system is another critical issue within the Black community, largely due to historical and ongoing experiences of discrimination and mistreatment. The notorious Tuskegee Syphilis Study, where Black men were deceived and denied treatment, is a prominent example of why many Black individuals remain wary of medical institutions. This mistrust can lead to delays in seeking care, lower adherence to medical advice, and poorer health outcomes. Building trust through culturally sensitive communication, community engagement, and patient-centered care is essential for improving healthcare outcomes in the Black community (Beach et al., 2006).

Lastly, the social determinants of health are crucial in understanding how community structures impact individual health outcomes. In Black communities, factors such as socioeconomic status, access to nutritious food, exposure to environmental hazards, and the availability of healthcare resources all play significant roles (Pronk et al., 2021).

For instance, the intersection of poverty, housing instability, and limited access to preventive healthcare services often leads to higher rates of chronic illnesses such as hypertension, diabetes, and heart disease. Clinicians need to consider these realities when treating patients from the Black community (Baciu et al., 2017).

CONCLUSION

The Black community is a rich and diverse mosaic, shaped by a wide range of cultural, historical, and sociological influences. Understanding the distinction between community and culture, and recognizing the impact of historical events like the African Diaspora and the Great Migration, is essential for fostering meaningful connections and delivering equitable obesity care. By acknowledging the complexity of Black communities, healthcare providers can offer more personalized and culturally responsive care, ultimately promoting better health outcomes for all.

CLINICAL CONSIDERATIONS CHECKLIST: WHAT IS THE "BLACK COMMUNITY?"

To translate this understanding into clinical practice, here is a quick checklist for clinicians when engaging with patients. Although this chapter focuses on the Black community, the questions can be used to assess community identity and values for individuals of all backgrounds.

Checklist Item	Recommendation	Clinical Question
I. Acknowledge Diversity The African Diaspora is very diverse. Black people may belong to several culturally distinct cultures and communities, including but not limited to: African American, Afro-Caribbean, African immigrant, and/or Afro-Latinx communities.	Recognize that the term "Black community" encompasses a wide range of identities and experiences. Avoid making assumptions based on appearance alone.	"Can you share with me anything about your background or identity that you feel is important for me to know as we work together on your health?"

(Continued)

Checklist Item	Recommendation	Clinical Question
2. Cultural Competence Matters Recognize and respect the cultural norms, beliefs, and practices of the Black community. Tailor healthcare interventions to align with these cultural factors, particularly in areas such as diet, physical activity, and mental health (Thorpe et al., 2021).	Invest time in learning about the cultural practices, communication styles, and healthcare beliefs that may be important to your patients.	"Are there any cultural practices, beliefs, or traditions that influence how you approach your healthcare or wellness?"
3. Be Aware of Systemic Barriers Address barriers to healthcare access that disproportionately affect the Black community, including economic challenges, lack of insurance, and geographic disparities. Advocate for policies that improve access to quality care for Black individuals (Bailey et al., 2017).	Understand the historical and sociological barriers that may affect your patients' healthcare access, such as economic instability, mistrust of medical institutions, or limited access to care.	"Have you faced any challenges or barriers in accessing healthcare that I should be aware of to better support you?"
4. Ask, Don't Assume Transparency and honest discussion are essential to avoid stereotypes based in historical racial bias.	When in doubt, ask patients about their experiences, preferences, and values. Personalized care is always better than relying on stereotypes.	"What are your preferences when it comes to your healthcare, and how can I best respect your values and priorities in our treatment plan?"
5. Self-Defined Community Leverage the social capital within Black communities, such as churches, community organizations, and social networks, to promote health and well-being. Engage community leaders and members in health promotion efforts (Holt et al., 2020).	Each individual may have a different definition of community, which may extend beyond superficial factors such as race. Invite individuals to define their own community rather than deciding for them.	"How would you define your community, and how do you feel it impacts your health and well-being?"

Chapter 3

Obesity as a Disease

Tiffani Bell-Washington, MD, MPH, MBA, FAPA,
FOMA, DABOM, DABLM,
Joynita R. Nicholson, DO, DABOM, FOMA, and
Sylvia Gonsahn-Bollie, MD, DABOM, FOMA

> Obesity is a multifactorial disorder with genetics, environment, develop-
> ment and behavior all playing a role, but a lot of people underemphasize
> genetics. We know that weight is more inheritable than height. If you have
> parents who have obesity the likelihood that the child will have obesity is
> really high, on the order of 50 to 85 percent likelihood, even with doing
> optimal behaviors, eating well, exercising.
>
> —Fatima Cody Stanford

Chapter 3 Highlights

- Obesity is a complex disease, not simply a lifestyle choice or due to a
  lack of willpower.
- The Body Mass Index (BMI) is not the best measure of individual obesity status. Black people are disproportionately impacted by the limitations of BMI.
- Understanding obesity requires an appreciation of historical, biological, and sociological factors, especially within the Black community.

INTRODUCTION

Obesity is a chronic, multifactorial disease, characterized by excess adipose
tissue accumulation, which significantly impacts nearly every system of the
human body, contributing to major health conditions such as diabetes, cardiovascular disease, and cancer. This chapter delves into the complexity of
obesity, emphasizing that it is not simply the result of individual lifestyle
choices but a disease influenced by genetic, biological, sociological, and environmental factors. Through an examination of the limitations of tools like
the Body Mass Index (BMI) and a focus on the unique challenges faced
by Black communities, this chapter highlights the need for comprehensive,
personalized approaches to obesity treatment. By exploring both the biological mechanisms and sociological determinants of obesity, this chapter sets

DOI: 10.1201/9781032622217-4

the foundation for understanding why targeted interventions that address social inequities and systemic barriers are essential for tackling the obesity epidemic.

FROM BELGIUM TO THE BODY MASS INDEX

Historically, obesity has been viewed as a lifestyle choice, influenced by misinformation and various forms of bias. In 2013, the American Medical Association (AMA) recognized obesity as a disease, highlighting the need for structured screening methods (American Medical Association, 2019). While the AMA recommends using waist circumference alongside Body Mass Index (BMI) for obesity screening, BMI remains the primary tool used in clinical settings. However, as discussed in Chapter 1, "Who Is Black?" BMI has notable limitations, particularly for Black individuals. Because BMI does not assess body composition, it cannot account for variations in muscle mass, bone density, or fat distribution, factors that differ across racial and ethnic groups and can lead to misclassification of health risks (Stanford, 2019).

The discrepancies in BMI may stem from its origins. Developed in the 1830s by Belgian mathematician Adolphe Quetelet, BMI was based on his observation that a person's weight changed in proportion to their height squared. In the 20th century, insurance companies adopted weight as a health indicator, recorded in "Life Tables," where "normal" weight standards were set by White men—the primary policyholders. In 1972, Dr. Ancel Keys, a physician and expert in body composition, sought to standardize weight as a health indicator, adopting Quetelet's calculation and naming it the Body Mass Index.

By 1985, both the U.S. National Institutes of Health and the World Health Organization had adopted BMI as a health measure (Strings, 2019a). By the 21st century, BMI became widely used in clinical settings, with the Centers for Medicare & Medicaid Services (CMS) implementing BMI as a quality-of-care measure, increasing pressure on clinicians to rely on BMI for health screening (Preventive Care and Screening: Body Mass Index [BMI] Screening and Follow-Up Plan, n.d.).

Sociologist Sabrina Strings argues that BMI reflects White European body standards and may perpetuate racial bias. She and researcher Lindo Bacon suggest that a focus on obesity and weight loss overlooks the impacts of racism and sexism on health outcomes (Strings, 2019). The devastating impacts of biases cannot be overlooked. Yet neither can obesity-related health risks that disproportionately affect Black individuals with higher morbidity and mortality rates related to obesity. A well-rounded obesity treatment plan should include considerations of nutrition, exercise, and medical options alongside social and historical factors uniquely affecting health in the Black community. Section III, "Opportunities" provides more details on creating comprehensive, culturally tailored obesity plans.

BIOLOGICAL ORIGINS OF OBESITY

Obesity is far more complex than the outdated notion of "calories in versus calories out." A consensus statement from six leading obesity organizations defines obesity as

> a highly prevalent chronic disease characterized by excessive fat accumulation or distribution that presents a risk to health and requires lifelong care. Virtually every system in the body is affected by obesity. Major chronic diseases associated with obesity include diabetes, heart disease, and cancer.

(George Washington University, STOP Obesity Alliance, 2024)

At its core, obesity results from an imbalance between energy intake and expenditure, but the pathways that control this balance involve numerous hormones, genetic predispositions, and brain signaling mechanisms.

One of the key biological factors that contributes to adipose stores is how the body regulates hunger and satiety through the orexigenic and anorexigenic pathways, respectively. Hormones such as ghrelin and leptin are central to this process. Examples of orexigenic hormones include ghrelin and peptide YY, while anorexigenic hormones include leptin, PYY and insulin (George & Guyenet, 2024). Ghrelin, often referred to as the "hunger hormone," stimulates appetite and is usually elevated before meals and suppressed afterward. In people with obesity, ghrelin may remain elevated, further promoting excessive food intake. Leptin, produced by fat cells, signals the brain when the body has sufficient energy stored, thereby reducing appetite. However, in people with obesity, this signaling can be disrupted—commonly referred to as leptin resistance—causing the brain to ignore these signals and leading to overeating (Tran et al., 2022).

The hypothalamus plays a central role in regulating energy balance by coordinating signals related to hunger and satiety. Within the brain region, two critical groups of neurons—the anorexigenic pro-opiomelanocortin (POMC) neurons and the orexigenic neurons producing neuropeptide Y (NPY) and agouti-related peptide (AgRP)—work in opposition to control appetite and energy expenditure. POMC neurons, which suppress appetite, release neuropeptides that activate melanocortin receptors, reducing food intake, regulating insulin levels, and promoting glucose balance. In contrast, NPY and AgRP neurons, located adjacent to POMC neurons, stimulate appetite by blocking POMC activity at downstream melanocortin receptors, thereby increasing food intake. This neuronal balance is heavily influenced by leptin and ghrelin signaling, with leptin inhibiting NPY/AgRP neurons and stimulating POMC neurons to reduce hunger. Disruptions in this system, such as leptin resistance seen in obesity, can impair the hypothalamus's ability to regulate hunger, leading to increased food intake and weight gain. Recent findings suggest that environmental and physiological factors modulate hypothalamic neurons' response to these signals, further complicating how hunger and satiety are regulated in obesity (George & Guyenet, 2024; Tran et al., 2022). This complex interplay underscores the importance of brain signaling mechanisms in obesity, revealing how hormonal imbalances and neural circuit disruptions contribute to the disease's persistence beyond lifestyle factors.

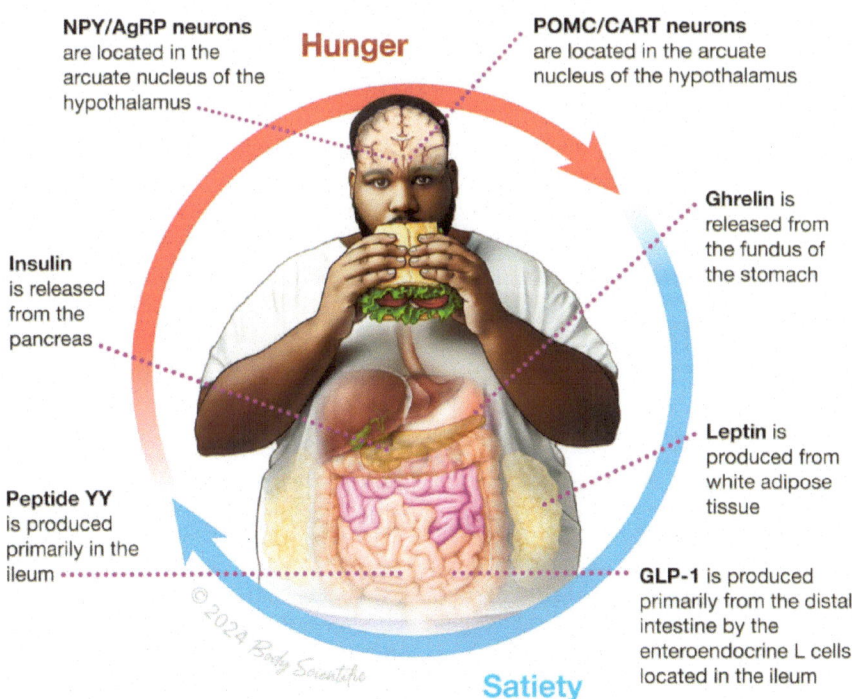

Hunger and Satiety Pathway

NPY/AgRP neurons are located in the arcuate nucleus of the hypothalamus

Hunger

POMC/CART neurons are located in the arcuate nucleus of the hypothalamus

Ghrelin is released from the fundus of the stomach

Insulin is released from the pancreas

Leptin is produced from white adipose tissue

Peptide YY is produced primarily in the ileum

GLP-1 is produced primarily from the distal intestine by the enteroendocrine L cells located in the ileum

Satiety

©2024 Body Scientific

In addition to hormonal regulation, genetics play a significant role in an individual's susceptibility to obesity. Studies have shown that specific genetic variants increase the likelihood of developing obesity. For example, the FTO gene, often referred to as the "fat mass and obesity-associated" gene, has been linked to higher body fat levels, increased appetite, and a reduced ability to feel full. Interestingly, the prevalence of certain obesity-related genetic variants is higher among Black populations. These genetic differences may influence how the body stores fat, responds to insulin, or manages energy expenditure, making it easier for some individuals to gain weight and harder for them to lose it (Byrd et al., 2018).

However, genetic predisposition alone does not fully explain the disparities in obesity rates across racial groups. Black communities face disproportionate levels of obesity, but environmental and social factors play a more significant role in amplifying these genetic risks. The interaction between genetic predispositions and environmental triggers, such as diet, stress, and physical activity levels, makes it difficult to attribute obesity to biological factors alone (Lofton et al., 2023).

Another critical biological component is the body's response to food intake through incretin hormones, such as glucagon-like peptide-1 (GLP-1) and gastric inhibitory polypeptide (GIP). GLP-1 slows digestion and promotes feelings of fullness, reducing food intake, while GIP regulates insulin release. Chapter 11, "Pharmacotherapy for Obesity Treatment," will discuss obesity treatments, including new-generation medications that mimic the effects of incretin hormones, which have recently gained prominence as highly effective treatments for obesity. These medications enhance the body's natural satiety signals, demonstrating that obesity treatment must address biological mechanisms, not just lifestyle modifications (Del Prato et al., 2022).

In summary, the biological origins of obesity underscore that it is not simply a matter of personal willpower or lifestyle choices. The interplay of hormones, genetics, and metabolic pathways makes obesity a complex disease requiring a multifaceted approach to treatment—one that considers both biological factors and societal influences that exacerbate these conditions in Black communities.

SOCIOLOGICAL ORIGINS OF OBESITY

Obesity is not just a biological condition; it is deeply rooted in societal structures, norms, and inequalities. The social determinants of health, such as socioeconomic status (SES), access to healthy food, the built environment, and cultural norms, significantly shape obesity prevalence, particularly in Black communities. Addressing these sociological factors is essential for developing effective interventions that go beyond individual behavior change.

Socioeconomic status is one of the most powerful predictors of obesity. People with lower SES often have limited access to healthy foods and safe spaces for physical activity. In many Black communities, "food deserts" are prevalent—urban or rural areas where residents have little access to affordable, nutritious food. These areas are often filled with fast-food outlets and convenience stores offering calorie-dense, processed foods, while fresh produce and lean proteins are hard to come by. This creates an environment where unhealthy eating habits are not just convenient but, for many, the only affordable option. In this context, obesity is not a failure of individual discipline but a reflection of systemic inequities (Cuevas et al., 2020).

The built environment also plays a significant role in shaping physical activity levels. Many Black communities lack access to parks, recreational facilities, and safe walking paths. High crime rates in certain neighborhoods further discourage outdoor activity, leaving residents with fewer opportunities to engage in exercise. Urban planning decisions often prioritize vehicular traffic over pedestrian access, promoting a sedentary lifestyle. Without safe, accessible spaces for physical activity, maintaining a healthy weight becomes increasingly difficult. These environmental barriers to exercise must be addressed in any public health initiative aimed at reducing obesity in Black communities.

Cultural norms also influence obesity rates. In some Black communities, larger body sizes have traditionally been associated with health, wealth, and beauty, offering protection against the stigma of thinness. Although these cultural values can act as a buffer against body-shaming, they may also complicate efforts to promote weight loss and healthy lifestyle changes. There is a delicate balance between respecting cultural differences and addressing the serious health risks posed by obesity, including diabetes, heart disease, and cancer. Effective interventions must navigate this cultural context thoughtfully and sensitively, promoting health without pathologizing body size.

Another critical sociological factor is the pervasive role of systemic racism. Systemic racism contributes to every factor discussed in this section, influencing access to resources, environmental conditions, and health outcomes. It also plays a significant role in shaping chronic stress experienced by many Black individuals due to ongoing racism and discrimination. This persistent stress triggers biological responses, such as the release of cortisol, which has been shown to increase appetite and promote fat storage, particularly in the abdominal area. When coupled with limited access to healthy coping mechanisms, this stress response creates a cycle that significantly contributes to obesity. The impact of systemic racism on both stress and overall health cannot be overlooked when addressing obesity in Black communities (Noonan et al., 2016).

Finally, the marketing of unhealthy foods disproportionately targets Black communities. Fast-food companies and sugary beverage manufacturers often direct their advertising efforts at low-income and minority populations, contributing to unhealthy dietary habits from a young age. This aggressive marketing, combined with limited nutrition education, further entrenches the cycle of obesity in Black communities. Efforts to combat obesity must therefore include not only individual education but also systemic changes in food marketing and access to healthy foods.

In summary, the sociological origins of obesity are intertwined with issues of access, equity, and cultural norms. To reduce obesity rates in Black communities, it is essential to address the root causes, such as food deserts, the built environment, cultural perceptions of body size, and the stress induced by systemic racism. Public health efforts that focus solely on personal responsibility or behavior change without tackling these broader societal issues will continue to fall short.

PUBLIC HEALTH IMPLICATIONS OF OBESITY

Obesity is not just a personal health issue; it is a significant public health concern with wide-reaching implications. The increasing prevalence of obesity, particularly in Black communities, poses serious challenges for public health systems. Addressing obesity requires a comprehensive approach that goes beyond individual behavior change to include broader societal interventions (Noonan et al., 2016).

One of the primary public health implications of obesity is its association with numerous chronic diseases. Obesity is a major risk factor for conditions such as type 2 diabetes, hypertension, cardiovascular disease, and certain cancers. These diseases are not only leading causes of death but also contribute to significant morbidity and healthcare costs. In Black communities, the burden of these obesity-related diseases is disproportionately high, exacerbating existing health disparities. For example, Black adults are nearly twice as likely as White adults to be diagnosed with diabetes, and this disparity is closely linked to higher obesity rates (Lofton et al., 2023; Noonan et al., 2016).

The economic impact of obesity is another critical public health concern. The costs associated with obesity are staggering, including direct medical expenses for treatment and indirect costs such as lost productivity and absenteeism. According to a study published in *Obesity Reviews*, the annual medical cost of obesity in the United States is estimated to be more than $147 billion, with higher costs in populations with higher obesity rates, including Black communities. These economic burdens strain public health resources and highlight the need for cost-effective interventions that can reduce the prevalence of obesity and its associated diseases (Centers for Disease Control and Prevention, 2009a).

Public health efforts to combat obesity must also address the social determinants of health, which are the conditions in which people are born, grow, live, work, and age. These determinants include factors such as socioeconomic status, education, neighborhood environments, and access to healthcare, all of which influence an individual's ability to maintain a healthy weight. Public health strategies that focus solely on individual behavior change, without addressing these broader determinants, are unlikely to be effective in reducing obesity rates (Lofton et al., 2023; Noonan et al., 2016).

Community-based interventions are a vital component of public health strategies to address obesity. These interventions can include initiatives to improve access to healthy foods, create safe spaces for physical activity, and provide education about nutrition and exercise. For example, programs that bring farmers' markets to urban neighborhoods or establish community gardens can increase access to fresh produce in areas where it is scarce. Similarly, public health campaigns that promote physical activity and provide resources for exercise can help combat sedentary lifestyles (Lofton et al., 2023).

Policy interventions are also crucial for addressing the public health implications of obesity. Policies that regulate the marketing of unhealthy foods, particularly to children, can help reduce the consumption of calorie-dense, nutrient-poor foods. Additionally, policies that support active transportation, such as biking and walking, can encourage physical activity and reduce obesity rates. Public health advocates can also push for policies that address the social determinants of health, such as increasing the minimum wage, improving access to education, and expanding healthcare coverage (Noonan et al., 2016).

The role of healthcare clinicians in addressing obesity is another important public health consideration. Clinicians need to be trained in culturally competent care to effectively treat obesity in Black communities. This includes understanding the unique challenges and barriers that individuals face, such as those related to socioeconomic status and cultural norms. Clinicians can also play a key role in early intervention by identifying patients at risk for obesity-related conditions and providing them with the resources and support they need to make healthy lifestyle changes (Lofton et al., 2023).

The public health implications of obesity are vast and complex, particularly within Black communities where the burden of disease is disproportionately high. Addressing obesity requires a multifaceted approach that includes individual behavior change, community-based interventions, policy changes, and culturally competent healthcare. By tackling the social determinants of health and implementing comprehensive public health strategies, we can begin to reduce the prevalence of obesity and improve health outcomes in Black communities.

CONCLUSION

Understanding obesity as a chronic, multifactorial disease requires moving beyond simplistic views of personal choice. This chapter has highlighted the historical, biological, sociological, and public health dimensions of obesity, illustrating how each factor contributes to the complexity of the disease. The limitations of BMI as a diagnostic tool, particularly for Black communities, underscore the need for more comprehensive and inclusive measures of health. Additionally, systemic barriers such as food deserts, limited access to safe spaces for physical activity, and the pervasive effects of racism create environments that increase obesity risk, especially among marginalized populations. Effective obesity treatment and prevention require a holistic approach that addresses both individual and societal factors, integrating personalized healthcare, policy changes, and community-based interventions. By tackling these underlying causes, we can develop more equitable and effective strategies to reduce obesity rates and improve health outcomes across diverse populations.

CLINICAL CONSIDERATIONS CHECKLIST: OBESITY AS A DISEASE

Obesity is a complicated disease with many causes. Research shows that racial and ethnic differences can sometimes lead to confusion in diagnosing obesity. This discussion guide is meant to help both patients and doctors by encouraging more accurate and personalized care, considering these differences. The following table provides a concise overview of key clinical considerations for assessing and managing obesity in Black populations. It includes relevant clinical questions for healthcare clinicians to facilitate patient-centered discussions during consultations.

Section	Key Considerations	Clinical Questions
1. Accuracy of BMI in Black Populations	BMI may not accurately reflect body fat percentage in Black individuals due to differences in muscle mass, bone density, and fat distribution.	• "Have you ever been told that your BMI might not accurately reflect your health status?" • "Are there other measures of health you would like us to consider, such as waist circumference or body fat percentage?"

(Continued)

Section	Key Considerations	Clinical Questions
2. Alternative Measures of Obesity	Consider using alternative measurements like waist circumference, waist-to-hip ratio, and body fat percentage. These may provide a better assessment of visceral fat and related health risks.	• "Would you be open to using other measures, such as waist circumference or a body composition analysis, to better understand your health risks?" • "How do you feel about using these alternative measures along with BMI?"
3. Sociocultural Perceptions of Body Size	Larger body sizes may be more culturally accepted or preferred in some Black communities, which can affect how patients perceive health risks and weight loss efforts.	• "How do you feel about your current weight and health?" • "What role do you feel cultural or family views play in your health goals?" • "What does being healthy mean to you?"
4. Historical and Systemic Factors	Systemic factors, such as access to healthcare, food deserts, and the stress from systemic racism, significantly impact obesity prevalence in Black communities.	• "Can you tell me about any challenges you face in accessing healthy foods or opportunities for exercise?" • "How do stress or other life experiences affect your health or weight?"
5. Genetic Predisposition	Genetic predispositions, such as variations in the FTO gene, may increase the risk of obesity in Black individuals, interacting with environmental factors.	• "Has anyone in your family struggled with weight-related health issues?" • "Are you aware of any genetic conditions that may impact your weight or health?"
6. Hormonal Regulation of Hunger and Satiety	Leptin resistance and abnormal ghrelin levels can influence hunger, satiety, and food intake in obesity.	• "Do you often feel hungry even after eating a meal?" • "Do you find that it's difficult to feel full or satisfied after eating?"
7. Role of Stress and Systemic Racism	Chronic stress from systemic racism can increase cortisol levels, contributing to abdominal fat accumulation and higher obesity risk.	• "How do stress and emotional well-being impact your eating or physical activity?" • "What kind of support would help you manage stress in a healthier way?"

(Continued)

(*Continued*)

Section	Key Considerations	Clinical Questions
8. Impact of Food Marketing and Availability	Marketing of unhealthy foods and limited access to nutritious options in predominantly Black communities perpetuate obesity.	• "Do you have access to fresh produce and healthy food options in your neighborhood?" • "Have you noticed an abundance of fast-food options where you live or work?"
9. Public Health Implications	Public health strategies must address social determinants, cultural sensitivity, and community engagement for sustainable weight management.	• "What community resources or supports would make it easier for you to achieve your health goals?" • "How can our healthcare team help connect you with resources to support a healthier lifestyle?"
10. Comprehensive and Personalized Treatment Plans	Treatment should be multifaceted, integrating biological, psychological, and sociocultural factors, and include medication, lifestyle modifications, and community support.®	• "What kind of support do you think would help you the most in reaching your health goals?" • "Are there any barriers to starting a weight management plan that we should address together?"

Section II

Obstacles

The Role of Social Determinants of Health on the Disease of Obesity

Kathi Earles, MD, MPH, DABOM and
Sylvia Gonsahn-Bollie, MD, DABOM, FOMA

> Health inequalities and the social determinants of health are not a foot-note to the determinants of health. They are the main issue.
>
> —Sir Michael Marmot

Chapter 4 Highlights

- **Social determinants** such as neighborhood conditions, education levels, and socioeconomic status significantly impact obesity rates, especially in marginalized Black and Brown communities. This environment fosters obesity-related factors that disproportionately affect these populations.
- **Shift workers** have a higher chance of overweight or obesity, with a 25% higher risk of being overweight and a 17% higher risk of obesity due to disrupted sleep and body rhythms (Liu et al., 2018; Gu et al., 2015).
- **Workplace wellness programs** can help reduce obesity and save money, lowering medical costs by $3.27 and reducing missed work costs by $2.73 for every dollar spent (Baicker et al., 2010).

INTRODUCTION

Despite the recognition of various factors contributing to the complex disease of obesity, the role of social determinants of health receives significantly less attention and intervention (Hahn, 2021; Riser et al., 2023). When factors such as neighborhood conditions, family income, education levels, and safety are acknowledged, actionable steps to reduce their impact often remain unaddressed (Krueger & Reither, 2015). Equally overlooked is the historical context that forced certain groups into economically, politically,

DOI: 10.1201/9781032622217-6

and socially marginalized communities, which have contributed to the high rates of obesity in these areas (Lovasi et al., 2009). This historical backdrop has created an environment rich in obesity-related causes, disproportionately affecting Black and Brown communities (Hahn, 2021). This chapter explores the systems that continue to exacerbate obesity disparities in marginalized communities (Krueger & Reither, 2015).

DEFINING SOCIAL DETERMINANTS OF HEALTH

Social determinants of health (SDOH) are the conditions in which people are born, grow, live, play, work, and age (Hahn, 2021). These conditions are shaped by the distribution of money, power, and resources at global, national, and local levels. Key SDOH relevant to obesity include socioeconomic status, education, physical environments, employment, social support networks, and access to comprehensive healthcare (Anekwe et al., 2020).

Historical Considerations and the Impact on Social Determinants of Health

Any discussion of obesity in marginalized communities must consider the history of systemic racism that laid the groundwork for today's disparities (Hahn, 2021). Globally, colonialism, apartheid, and other forms of systemic racism have contributed to health inequities (Riser et al., 2023). For example, in the United States, the impact of the Serviceman's Readjustment Act of 1944 (the GI Bill) played a significant role in post–Civil War inequities (Eden, 2023). This legislation aimed to reward military service with opportunities for low-interest loans, education, and unemployment benefits (Eden, 2023). The GI Bill was intended to elevate veterans into the middle class, providing a path toward postwar prosperity (Eden, 2023). However, the benefits were not distributed equally, with Black veterans receiving significantly less access to education and financial opportunities compared to their White counterparts (Riser et al., 2023). This inequality was even more pronounced in the South compared to the North (Eden, 2023). The result was an exacerbation of Black–White gaps in education and economic opportunities (Krueger & Reither, 2015). Black veterans who could access educational benefits were often limited to trade schools rather than 4-year colleges (Eden, 2023). Furthermore, when Black veterans did qualify for home loans, they were often restricted from purchasing homes in affluent White neighborhoods that provided access to essential resources such as grocery stores, green spaces, healthcare, and quality education (Eden, 2023; Krueger & Reither, 2015). This history of racial discrimination laid the foundation for decades of health disparities in Black communities (Krueger & Reither, 2015).

SOCIOECONOMIC STATUS AND OBESITY

A strong link exists between socioeconomic status (SES) and obesity, with lower SES often associated with higher obesity rates (Anekwe et al., 2020). Discrimination due to race and ethnicity have historically limited access to education, occupational advancement, income, and wealth, further contributing to health disparities (Krueger & Reither, 2015). Financial insecurity in marginalized communities has led to the creation of food deserts, increased exposure to violence, and reduced opportunities for physical activity (Mohammed et al., 2019). Families in these communities often purchase cheaper, calorie-dense foods due to financial constraints, further contributing to obesity (Krueger & Reither, 2015). Research consistently shows that individuals from lower socioeconomic backgrounds face higher exposure to obesity-promoting environments compared to their wealthier counterparts (Anekwe et al., 2020). Simply living in a low-SES neighborhood has been linked to higher risks of overweight and obesity, regardless of an individual's personal SES (Mohammed et al., 2019). These obesity-promoting environments negatively impact residents, although the effects differ between men and women (Krueger & Reither, 2015). Women with lower SES tend to have higher obesity rates inversely related to income, whereas men have a positive correlation between income and body mass index (BMI) (Krueger & Reither, 2015). Addressing these challenges requires altering the built environment to encourage physical activity and healthy eating (Anekwe et al., 2020). Creating safe places to exercise, increasing access to full-service grocery stores, limiting the marketing of unhealthy foods, and improving neighborhood safety can promote healthier lifestyles (Mohammed et al., 2019). Research shows that time spent in cars is linked to obesity, with a 3% increase in risk for every 30 additional minutes spent driving (Frank et al., 2004). Community design, including walkability, green spaces, and sidewalks is directly associated with residents' physical activity levels (Frank et al., 2004).

EDUCATION

Educational attainment is closely tied to obesity outcomes (Sart et al., 2023). Higher education levels are associated with better health literacy, which is crucial for making informed health decisions (Finley, 2023). Research shows that education influences obesity in multiple ways, serving as a key factor in economic growth and personal income (Sart et al., 2023). Higher education also increases awareness of the determinants of obesity and associated health risks (Zajacova & Lawrence, 2021). Furthermore, individuals with higher education have better access to information about healthcare services and healthy living (Zajacova & Lawrence, 2021). The relationship between education and obesity varies between genders, with lower education linked more strongly to obesity in women than in men (Sart et al., 2023). Men with lower education tend to have higher rates of total obesity, whereas women show a stronger association with both total and central obesity (Sart et al., 2023).

PHYSICAL ENVIRONMENT

Extensive research shows a connection between the built environment and obesity rates in both children and adults (Lovasi et al., 2009). Factors such as the lack of green space, sidewalks, grocery stores with healthy options, and recreational centers, as well as the prevalence of fast-food outlets, crime, and poverty, all contribute to increased obesity rates (Townshend & Lake, 2017). However, less attention is given to the physical environment and how it affects social interactions within communities, thereby also influencing obesity (Lovasi et al., 2009). Diez-Roux and Mair (2010) define the social environment as the socio-demographic composition of a neighborhood and the social relationships and processes that occur between residents. Social cohesion, social capital, norms, collective efficacy, crime rates, poverty, and segregation are all factors that shape the social environment (Diez-Roux & Mair, 2010). Poverty and high crime rates are associated with a lack of social cohesion, contributing to the development of obesogenic environments (Alhasan et al., 2023). In neighborhoods with low social cohesion, obesity rates are 20% higher in women and 10% higher in men compared to neighborhoods with greater social cohesion (Alhasan et al., 2023).

EMPLOYMENT AND WORK CONDITIONS

Shift workers comprise approximately 15% of the workforce nationwide. Men, minorities, and individuals with lower education are more commonly shift workers (Saulle et al., 2018). Minorities and individuals with lower education also show one of the highest prevalences of obesity (Saulle et al., 2018). A study by Liu et al. (2018) analyzed 27 studies involving more than 300,000 shift workers and found a positive association between shift work and the risk of obesity or being overweight. The study assessed various shift work schedules, including night shifts and rotating shifts, showing a 25% and 17% increase in the prevalence of overweight and obesity, respectively (Liu et al., 2018).

One mechanism believed to contribute to this increase is the disruption of normal sleep patterns, blood glucose regulation, energy metabolism, and inflammation, all of which intensify the risk of obesity (Gu et al., 2015). It has also been linked to the desynchronization of an employee's physiological rhythm (Gu et al., 2015). This desynchronization impacts daily activities, such as eating habits, circadian rhythms, and physical activity (D'Ettorre et al., 2019). A subsequent study by Gu and colleagues (2015) demonstrated that even temporary adjustments in sleep patterns might increase the risk of cardiovascular disease and overall mortality by 11%. Another study involving male and female nurses without metabolic syndrome at the study's start followed participants annually for 4 years. By the end of the study, the cumulative incidence rate of metabolic syndrome was 9% in night shift workers compared to 1.8% in daytime workers (Gu et al., 2015). Further research showed that visceral adiposity in night shift workers was 14% compared to 7.7% in daytime workers after 4 years (Gu et al., 2015).

These studies illustrate the association between shift work and obesity. However, workplace wellness programs and encouraging physical activity can help mitigate these risks (Baicker et al., 2010). Workplace wellness programs have been shown to not only improve employee mental and physical health but also reduce company healthcare costs (Baicker et al., 2010). For instance, an analysis of several studies assessing the financial benefits of wellness programs found that medical costs decreased by approximately $3.27 for every dollar spent on such programs, while absenteeism costs were reduced by $2.73 for every dollar spent (Baicker et al., 2010). Addressing both the quality and quantity of work while implementing strategies to reverse obesity trends is crucial in managing the rising prevalence of obesity among shift workers (Baicker et al., 2010).

SOCIAL SUPPORT AND HEALTHCARE ACCESS

Social support networks play a pivotal role in influencing health behaviors related to obesity. A supportive social environment encourages healthy eating and physical activity (Hahn, 2021). Access to healthcare allows for the timely intervention and management of diseases, including obesity (Buchmueller et al., 2016). The Affordable Care Act (ACA) provisions in 2014 led to a significant decline in the percentage of uninsured adults (Buchmueller et al., 2016). Hispanic, Black, and White populations saw reductions of 7.1%, 5.1%, and 3%, respectively (Buchmueller et al., 2016). Coverage gains were particularly notable in states that expanded Medicaid programs with ACA funds (Buchmueller et al., 2016). States with higher obesity rates, particularly those that did not accept ACA funds, are often heavily populated by Black and Brown residents (Buchmueller et al., 2016). Accepting ACA funds has been associated with improved healthcare access for these communities, which are disproportionately affected by obesity and related comorbidities (Buchmueller et al., 2016).

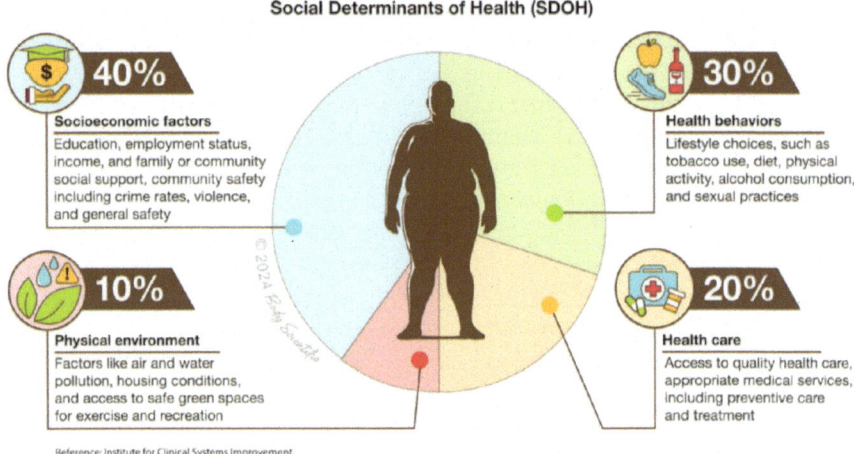

Social Determinants of Health (SDOH)

40%
Socioeconomic factors
Education, employment status, income, and family or community social support, community safety including crime rates, violence, and general safety

30%
Health behaviors
Lifestyle choices, such as tobacco use, diet, physical activity, alcohol consumption, and sexual practices

10%
Physical environment
Factors like air and water pollution, housing conditions, and access to safe green spaces for exercise and recreation

20%
Health care
Access to quality health care, appropriate medical services, including preventive care and treatment

Reference: Institute for Clinical Systems Improvement.
Going Beyond Clinical Walls: Solving Complex Problems (October 2014)

CONCLUSION AND FUTURE DIRECTIONS

The influence of social determinants on obesity is undeniable and multifaceted (Hahn, 2021). Addressing obesity requires a comprehensive approach that takes into account the social and environmental contexts in which individuals live (Riser et al., 2023). Public health interventions must focus not only on individual behaviors but also on creating supportive environments that facilitate healthy choices (Hahn, 2021). Future research should explore additional mechanisms through which social determinants affect obesity and identify interventions that can mitigate these impacts (Riser et al., 2023).

Moving forward, collaboration among healthcare providers, policymakers, community leaders, and patients is essential in tackling the obesity epidemic (Hahn, 2021). By addressing social determinants of health, we can work toward a future where all individuals have the opportunity to achieve and maintain optimal, equitable health and wellness (Hahn, 2021).

CLINICAL CONSIDERATIONS CHECKLIST: SOCIAL DETERMINANTS OF HEALTH IN OBESITY MANAGEMENT DISCUSSION

This guide facilitates a conversation between clinicians and patients about the critical role that social determinants of health (SDOH) play in the disease of obesity. By understanding these factors, patients can identify personal challenges and collaborate with their healthcare providers to develop actionable strategies for improved health outcomes.

Discussion Points	Questions/Notes
Understanding SDOH	• What are the key social determinants in your life?
	• How do they impact your health and lifestyle?
Impact of SDOH on Obesity	• How do neighborhood conditions affect your eating and activity levels?
	• In what ways has your education influenced your health choices?
Historical Context	• What historical factors do you believe impact your health today?
	• How do systemic issues affect your community's health?
Work Conditions and Health	• Do you have experience with shift work? How does it affect your health?
	• Are there wellness programs at your workplace?
Social Support and Healthcare Access	• Who supports you in your health journey?
	• Have you faced any barriers in accessing healthcare?
Actionable Steps	• Identify one social determinant you can address (e.g., improve access to healthy foods, engage in community support).
	• Discuss community resources that could help address SDOH related to obesity (e.g., local food banks, exercise programs).
Follow-Up	• Schedule follow-up appointments to discuss progress and any new barriers encountered.
Conclusion	• Reflect on how SDOH affects your health and consider solutions with your healthcare provider.

Weight Bias and Cultural Attitudes toward Obesity

Sylvia Gonsahn-Bollie, MD, DABOM, FOMA,
Kathi Earles, MD, MPH, DABOM, and
Tiffani Bell-Washington, MD, MPH, MBA, FAPA,
FOMA, DABOM, DABLM

> All weight bias does is trap people in a spiral of shame and self-blame, neither of which works to address the very real, medical problem of obesity.
>
> —Nikki Massie, Obesity Advocate
> Obesity Action Coalition Board Member

Chapter 5 Highlights

- **Addressing Weight Bias:** Weight bias, both external and internalized, disproportionately affects minorities and women, influencing healthcare experiences and perpetuating stigma. Acknowledging and dismantling this bias is essential for holistic obesity care.
- **Cultural Norms and Beauty Standards:** Black beauty standards often celebrate fuller body types, contrasting with mainstream ideals that glorify thinness. Understanding these cultural differences helps clinicians offer more respectful and effective obesity management.
- **Culturally Tailored Motivational Interviewing:** Healthcare clinicians should use culturally sensitive approaches, such as motivational interviewing, to help patients set personal, realistic health goals that align with their cultural values and promote overall well-being.

INTRODUCTION

Cultural attitudes toward obesity play a significant role in how individuals perceive their bodies and manage their health. This chapter examines these cultural perspectives, particularly in the Black community, and explores how weight bias, beauty standards, and cultural norms impact obesity care. It emphasizes the importance of understanding and addressing weight bias, both external and internalized, and advocates for a culturally sensitive, holistic approach to obesity management. By recognizing these cultural attitudes

DOI: 10.1201/9781032622217-7

and offering individualized care, healthcare clinicians can create more effective and respectful strategies for managing obesity, supporting patients in achieving their health goals without stigmatizing their body size.

WEIGHT BIAS: INTERNALIZED AND EXTERNALIZED

Weight bias refers to discrimination or negative attitudes directed at individuals based on their body size. Some may refer to it as "fatphobia," but in medical contexts "weight bias" is the preferred term, as the former is considered outdated. Regardless of the nomenclature, weight bias is common, even in healthcare settings. According to the Obesity Action Coalition, 29% of African Americans report experiencing weight bias in healthcare settings (OAC Online Survey, 2020). This bias can be external, originating from societal attitudes, or internalized, where individuals adopt negative beliefs about their own bodies. Explicit bias is when someone knowingly holds and expresses unfair beliefs about a group, whereas implicit bias happens automatically without the person realizing it (Pearl & Puhl, 2018).

Those most vulnerable to weight bias include individuals with larger bodies, minorities, and women, who often face compounded discrimination due to both gender bias and racism. Statistics highlighting that Black women have the highest rates of overweight and obesity often neglect the added psychological toll of weight bias. Although some Black women may culturally embrace a curvier body type, many are influenced by mainstream beauty standards that promote thinness as the ideal. This internalization is often reinforced by exposure to obesity-related health issues within families, leading to the adoption of these negative attitudes.

Despite the high prevalence of weight bias, research shows that non-Hispanic Black patients are less likely to avoid healthcare out of fear of weight discussions. A 2016 study by Lewis and colleagues found that Black patients were more open than their White counterparts to discussing weight-related treatment options (Lewis et al., 2016). Clinicians should remain aware of the compounded impact of biases when treating Black patients. However, this awareness should not deter sensitive discussions of care options, provided they are respectful of individual preferences.

Comprehensive obesity treatment extends beyond weight loss, encompassing both mental and physical health. Individual wellness goals are integrated to ensure a personalized treatment plan that aligns with the patient's unique lifestyle. Solutions for addressing weight bias in healthcare settings will be discussed later in this chapter, with further details provided in Chapter 9, "Behavioral Impact and Interventions in the Treatment of Obesity." Additionally, a weight-centric focus during healthcare visits can result in missed opportunities to address other medical concerns, ultimately worsening outcomes for patients with obesity (Fulton et al., 2023).

Black Beauty Standards vs. Mainstream Beauty Standards

Beauty standards, deeply embedded in cultural norms, shape how individuals perceive themselves and others. In the United States, mainstream beauty ideals—largely shaped by media and fashion industries—tend to glorify thin, often unrealistic body types for the average person. These ideals can lead to widespread body dissatisfaction and reinforce the stigma associated with obesity.

In contrast, Black beauty standards often celebrate fuller body types. Historically, within Black culture, a larger body size has been linked to attributes such as health, wealth, and fertility. This cultural perspective offers a protective shield against the negative body image issues perpetuated by mainstream standards, fostering a sense of pride and confidence in one's appearance (Agyemang & Powell-Wiley, 2013).

However, the gap between Black beauty standards and mainstream ideals can create tension. Black individuals may feel pressured to conform to societal expectations that conflict with their cultural identity. This is especially true for Black women, who often find themselves navigating complex beauty standards that may not align with their cultural values or physical characteristics (Robinson et al., 2020).

BODY SIZE AND BODY INCLUSIVITY

The body positivity movement, which promotes the acceptance and appreciation of all body types, has gained significant momentum in recent years. This movement resonates deeply within the Black community, where larger body sizes are often embraced as symbols of cultural pride and beauty.

Body positivity challenges harmful narratives that equate thinness with health and worth, encouraging individuals to value their bodies as they are. For many Black women, body positivity is about reclaiming control over their bodies and resisting societal pressures to conform to narrow beauty standards (Strings, 2019).

Body inclusivity honors the diversity of body types, acknowledging that health and well-being can exist across a range of sizes (Bryan, 2024). This philosophy should not be confused with the Fat Acceptance Movement (FAM) Health at Every Size (HAES) movement, or the National Association to Advance Fat Acceptance [NAAFA], 2024; Association for Size Diversity and Health [ASDAH], 2024). Although these organizations serve vital roles within their communities, their discussion lies beyond the scope of this chapter, as HAES does not prioritize and NAAFA does not acknowledge obesity as a disease.

In the media, body positivity and body inclusivity are often framed as being at odds with obesity care. In reality, many of their core principles—such as self-compassion, respect for others, and valuing diverse body types—are integral to holistic, individualized obesity care. These principles align with the goal of supporting health while fostering self-acceptance and respect for all body types.

Balancing Body Inclusivity and Health Goals in Care

Healthcare clinicians can promote body inclusivity by addressing implicit bias and recognizing that health exists across a range of body shapes and weights. Shifting the focus from weight loss to health outcomes and lifestyle changes can help reduce the negative psychological impacts of weight bias. By promoting body acceptance and healthier habits without the stigma of weight, clinicians can foster stronger, more supportive relationships with patients.

Body inclusivity is a powerful tool for promoting self-esteem and combating stigma, but it's essential to balance acceptance with a focus on health. Clinicians should support these principles while guiding patients toward healthier lifestyles. Although body weight management is a key component of obesity treatment, it is only one part of a comprehensive care plan. Section III, "Opportunities," will explore the goals of culturally tailored obesity care and potential treatment options.

The objective of obesity care is not to impose weight loss. Instead, it seeks to empower patients to make informed decisions that enhance their health and well-being, regardless of body size (Puhl et al., 2016).

DETERMINING "HAPPY WEIGHT"

The concept of a "happy weight" refers to the weight at which an individual feels comfortable, healthy, and content. This weight isn't necessarily the lowest possible or one that aligns with societal standards, but rather the point where the person feels their best both physically and emotionally. Unlike "healthy weight," which is based on clinical assessments, happy weight is rooted in self-perception (Gonsahn-Bollie, 2021).

Determining a happy weight is a deeply personal process. For some, it may involve losing weight to alleviate health issues, whereas for others, it may mean embracing a higher weight with cultural or personal significance. In the Black community, where larger body sizes are often celebrated, happy weight may represent a balance between cultural values and health goals (Fletcher et al., 2021).

Although individuals determine their own happy weight, weight bias can sometimes distort self-perception. Clinicians play a crucial role in helping patients identify their true happy weight through motivational interviewing and guided self-reflection (Gonsahn-Bollie, 2021). This process should be collaborative, with clinicians actively listening to and respecting patients' goals and values. The focus should remain on health and well-being rather than solely on weight loss. Encouraging patients to set realistic, sustainable goals that prioritize how they feel over how they look can lead to positive, lasting outcomes (Mensinger et al., 2018). Additionally, the process of discussing weight perception may reveal previous trauma or untreated psychological conditions, and clinicians should be prepared to refer patients to appropriate professionals for care. See Chapter 9, "Behavioral Impact and Interventions in the Treatment of Obesity," for more information on the connection between mental health and obesity care.

CULTURALLY TAILORED MOTIVATIONAL INTERVIEWING

Motivational interviewing (MI) is a counseling approach designed to help individuals resolve ambivalence about change and strengthen their motivation to adopt healthier behaviors. When working within the Black community, it is essential that MI be culturally tailored to reflect the values, beliefs, and experiences of Black patients.

Culturally tailored MI goes beyond simply translating words; it requires a deep understanding of the cultural context in which a patient lives. This includes recognizing the cultural significance of certain foods, understanding the role of family and community in decision-making, and acknowledging experiences with racism and healthcare bias (Miller, 2023).

In practice, healthcare clinicians should engage in conversations that are empathetic, non-judgmental, and culturally aware. They should ask openended questions that allow patients to express their values and concerns and listen actively to understand the patient's perspective. This approach helps patients identify their own motivations for change and develop strategies that align with their cultural identity and personal goals (Miller & Rollnick, 2021).

Actionable Steps

- **Dismantling Weight Bias:** Support campaigns such as the STOP Weight Bias initiative by the Obesity Action Coalition and the Rudd Center for Food Policy and Health, which aim to combat weight stigma and provide education on the harmful effects of weight bias.

- **Increase Awareness of Clinician Bias:** Encourage healthcare clinicians to reflect on their implicit biases by taking tools like the Harvard Implicit Association Test on weight, helping to identify subconscious biases and promote equitable treatment.

- **Train Healthcare Clinicians on Cultural Competency:** Incorporate mandatory training on cultural competency and weight bias for both practicing clinicians and those in training. This helps current and future clinicians recognize, address, and mitigate their biases while fostering more empathetic communication with patients from diverse backgrounds. Such training not only improves communication but also promotes better health outcomes.

- **Promote Body Inclusivity alongside Health Education:** Promote body inclusivity in healthcare by recognizing that health exists across a range of body sizes. Shifting healthcare goals from weight loss to a broader focus on health outcomes and well-being reduces the negative psychological impacts of weight bias. This approach fosters stronger patient–clinician relationships and supports long-term health.

- **Integrate Culturally Tailored Motivational Interviewing:** Equip healthcare clinicians with motivational interviewing techniques that respect cultural differences. This involves active listening, understanding cultural values, and helping patients set realistic, personal health goals that prioritize overall well-being.

- **Develop Community-Based Obesity Prevention Programs:** Work with local leaders and organizations within Black and minority communities to create culturally relevant wellness and obesity prevention programs. These programs should be accessible and address the unique socioeconomic and cultural challenges these groups face.

- **Shift to Comprehensive Care:** Move away from weight-centric care models and focus on holistic well-being, addressing both physical and mental health. This approach helps ensure that medical concerns unrelated to weight are not overlooked, improving overall health outcomes.

- **Create Safe and Inclusive Healthcare Environments:** Advocate for training and policies that reduce bias within healthcare systems. Building an inclusive and respectful healthcare environment can help patients of all body sizes and backgrounds feel valued and supported.

CONCLUSION

In conclusion, Chapter 5, "Weight Bias and Cultural Attitudes toward Obesity," highlights the essential role that cultural norms, weight bias, and beauty standards play in shaping the obesity experience, particularly within the Black community. The chapter calls for a culturally sensitive approach to obesity care that prioritizes holistic health instead of weight-centric care. Through understanding cultural attitudes and implementing comprehensive, empathetic healthcare, clinicians can more effectively address both the physical and psychological aspects of obesity, leading to better patient outcomes. Solutions to weight bias will be further explored in the Behavioral Health chapter, offering additional strategies to combat this pervasive issue.

CLINICAL CONSIDERATIONS CHECKLIST: SETTING COLLABORATIVE OBESITY GOALS

Setting obesity goals with patients requires a collaborative approach, cultural sensitivity, and a focus on the patient's overall well-being. The following Interactive Conversation Guide for Clinicians and Patients contains key considerations for healthcare clinicians working with Black patients to set collaborative obesity goals.

Conversation Stage	Clinical Action	Sample Questions or Prompts
One: Start with the Patient's Perspective	• Ask open-ended questions about the patient's goals, values, and concerns. • Explore what a healthy lifestyle means to them and how their cultural background affects them.	• "What does a healthy lifestyle look like for you?" • "How do your cultural values shape your health goals?"
Two: Focus on Health, Not Just Weight	• Discuss health goals beyond weight loss, such as improving activity levels, eating a balanced diet, and managing stress. • Reframe weight loss as one of the potential benefits, not the primary objective.	• "What goals besides weight loss would you like to focus on?" • "How can we work together to reduce stress and improve your well-being?"
Three: Respect Cultural Values	• Acknowledge the cultural significance of body size within the Black community. • Collaborate with the patient to balance cultural pride with health goals (e.g., modifying traditional recipes while maintaining cultural meaning).	• "How can we balance your cultural traditions with your health goals?" • "Are there traditional foods we can modify to be healthier?"
Four: Encourage Realistic and Sustainable Goals	• Work with the patient to set small, realistic, and sustainable goals. • Focus on gradual changes that fit their lifestyle, and find activities they enjoy to promote well-being.	• "What small changes can you make that feel manageable?" • "What physical activities do you enjoy?"

(Continued)

(Continued)

Conversation Stage	Clinical Action	Sample Questions or Prompts
Five: Provide Ongoing Support	• Provide ongoing encouragement through follow-ups, either in-person or digitally. • Adjust goals as necessary based on progress, and offer support for challenges the patient may encounter.	• "How are you feeling about your progress so far?" • "Would you prefer in-person follow-ups or virtual check-ins?"
Six: Build Trust	• Be transparent and respectful in all interactions. • Address any mistrust the patient may have toward the healthcare system and build confidence through culturally sensitive, compassionate care.	• "What has your experience with the healthcare system been like?" • "How can I support you in feeling more comfortable during our visits?"

By approaching obesity management with cultural competence and a collaborative mindset, healthcare clinicians can empower Black patients to achieve their health goals in a way that respects their cultural identity and personal values.

Chapter 6

Clinical Assessment and the Disease of Obesity

Kathi Earles, MD, MPH, DABOM,
Sylvia Gonsahn-Bollie, MD, DABOM, FOMA, and
Marci Bennafield, MPH

Listening to patients is the cornerstone of patient-centered care.

—Don Berwick, Former Administrator
Centers for Medicare & Medicaid Services

Chapter 6 Highlights

- Providing a comprehensive clinical assessment in a compassionate and empathetic manner is a necessary component to lay the groundwork for improved patient outcomes.
- Addressing and rectifying bias and stigma toward patients with obesity perpetrated throughout the healthcare setting is an essential component toward achieving optimum patient care outcomes. Bias is compounded in Black patients with obesity.
- A detailed clinical assessment designed to secure information regarding the patient's history, risk assessment, and motivation for change is a key feature in achieving optimum healthcare outcomes.

INTRODUCTION

Globally, 2.2 billion people, 42% of the world's population, are overweight or have obesity based on a body mass index (BMI) of >25 kg/m². In the United States (U.S.), according to the latest information released by the U.S. Centers for Disease Control and Prevention (CDC), more than 40% of American adults, ages 20 and older, have a BMI >30 kg/m², consistent with the definition of obesity as defined by the World Health Organization (Brown et al., 2022). Adults ages 40–59 years were noted to have the highest obesity prevalence at 46.4%, slightly 10% and 12% greater than the prevalence in adults ages 20–39 years and 60 years and older, respectively. The obesity prevalence is anticipated to reach 50% for all adults by the year 2030 (Ward et al., 2019).

DOI: 10.1201/9781032622217-8

A thorough clinical assessment of patients with overweight and obesity is a vital component to developing a patient-centered treatment plan designed to facilitate weight reduction and mitigate the associated comorbidities.

CLINICAL ASSESSMENT

In the traditional paternalistic model, the physician made all of the healthcare decisions without the endorsement from the patient (Jaffee & Christian, 2019). This unequal power dynamic often resulted in a suboptimal relationship between the clinician and the patient, which negatively impacted patient care and health outcomes. Present methods of healthcare delivery rely upon shared decision-making between the patient and clinician. Shared decision-making is the patient and clinician working together as a team. The first clinician and patient interaction is the foundation for establishing a healthy environment based upon compassion and a commitment to achieving optimal health outcomes.

Motivational Interviewing

Motivational interviewing is a collaborative, person-centered counseling approach that can be used during shared decision-making. The aim of motivational interviewing is to enhance the individual's intrinsic motivation by focusing on their own goals, values, and reasons to change (Bischof et al., 2021).

The steps outlined in motivational interviewing, shown in Clinical Considerations Checklist at the end of the chapter, cultivate a safe space where the patient can describe their goals and the patient and clinician can construct a blueprint for success together. The blueprint begins with education on the disease of obesity delivered in a clear and compassionate manner. A key component of the discussion is to emphasize the complexity of obesity as a disease influenced by a multitude of factors beyond the control of the patient. It can be a relief to hear that "Obesity is not your fault." An empathetic and informative dialogue will contribute to eliminating years of self-blame and encourage movement toward weight loss directed at improving physical and mental health. Please see the table in Clinical Considerations on tips for motivational interviewing.

CLINICAL ASSESSMENT FOR ADDRESSING AND DEVELOPING A PLAN FOR TREATMENT

A thorough clinical assessment that includes a comprehensive history, physical examination, and laboratory test serves as the cornerstone for the development of an effective obesity treatment plan (Mallik et al., 2023). The treatment plan should comprehensively address the patient's unique biological, psychological, and social contributors to obesity. Table 6.1 outlines the key components of an effective, individualized obesity assessment and treatment.

Table 6.1 Key Components of an Effective, Individualized Obesity Assessment and Treatment

Category	Assessment Criteria	Key Considerations
Patient History	Medical History Weight History	• Obtain past medical history, including birth history. • Review history of weight gain; identify potential weight gain triggers. • Review previous attempts at weight loss including past use of anti-obesity medications, bariatric procedures, diets, or eating plans.
	Family History	• Family history of obesity, diabetes, CVD, metabolic disease, cancers, mental health history.
	Psychological History	• Evaluate for depression, anxiety, stress, disordered eating.
	Medications	• Assess for medications contributing to weight gain, including antidepressants, steroids, beta-blockers, etc.
	Sleep Patterns	• Assess for sleep disorders such as sleep apnea, inadequate sleep duration, and decreased quality of quality of sleep.
	Physical Activity	• Determine level, type, and frequency of physical activity or level of physical inactivity.
	Dietary History	• Assess eating habits, portion sizes, meal frequency, and types of food consumed.
Physical Examination	Body Mass Index	• Calculate BMI (kg/m^2); use adjusted, culturally specific BMI charts for Black and Hispanic patients for comparison.
	Waist Circumference	• Measure waist circumference comparing with appropriate values for age and ethnicity.
	Blood Pressure	• Measure resting blood pressure to screen for hypertension.
	Dermatological Signs of Insulin Resistance	• Check for acanthosis nigricans or skin tags.
	Thyroid Examination	• Palpate for thyroid enlargement, nodules, or tenderness.
	Joint Examination	• Evaluate for joint tenderness, crepitus, or swelling associated with excess weight +/− osteoarthritis.

(Continued)

Table 6.1   (Continued)

Category	Assessment Criteria	Key Considerations
Laboratory Tests	Fasting Blood Glucose/ HbA1c	• Screen for diabetes or prediabetes.
	Lipid Panel	• Assess cholesterol levels, LDL, HDL, triglycerides.
	Liver Function Test	• Evaluate for elevated AST/ALT, which may suggest metabolic dysfunction associated liver disease (MAFLD)—> RUQ ultrasound indicated for diagnosis.
	Thyroid Function Tests	• Assess for hypothyroidism (TSH, free, T4).
	Other Hormonal Tests	• Assess cortisol, testosterone, and insulin levels as appropriate.
Associated Health Conditions and Risk Assessment	Cardiovascular Vascular Health (CVH) and Cardiovascular Disease (CVD) Risk	• Utilize composite scores from American Heart Association such as Life's Essential 8 Score for CVH or PREVENT for CVD risk.
	Type 2 Diabetes Risk	• Evaluate based on family history, fasting glucose, and HbA1c.
	Obstructive Sleep Apnea	• Use screening tools such as the STOP-BANG Questionnaire; assess for snoring or daytime sleepiness.
Behavioral and Psychological	Eating Disorders/ Disordered Eating	• Assess for binge eating disorder, atypical anorexia nervosa, bulimia nervosa, food addiction, dieting, or emotional eating.
	Motivation for Long-Term Obesity Care (sustainable weight loss and health optimization)	• Discuss the patient's readiness for behavior change and learnings from previous weight management strategies.
	Mental Health Status	• Screen for anxiety (GAD-7), depression (PHQ-9), or other mood disorders using DSM-V.
Treatment	Behavioral Changes	• Develop individualized goals for behavior therapy, dietary changes, and physical activity.
	Pharmacotherapy	• Consider anti-obesity medications based on BMI, medical conditions, family history, and patient preferences/ lifestyle needs.

(Continued)

Table 6.1 Key Components of an Effective, Individualized Obesity Assessment and Treatment (*Continued*)

Category	Assessment Criteria	Key Considerations
Treatment (Contd)	Surgical Options	• Evaluate eligibility for bariatric surgery if indicated.
	Referral to Specialist	• Refer to dietician, obesity medicine specialist/bariatrician, endocrinologist, behavioral health clinician, or other specialist as needed.
Follow-Up and Monitoring	Regular Follow-Up (should be monthly for at least 6 months, then every 3 months)	• Schedule follow-ups for treatment monitoring, goal adjustment, and support.
	Reassess Comorbidities	• Monitor diabetes, cardiovascular, and other related conditions.
	Evaluate Treatment Efficacy	• Assess progress with current interventions and adjust if necessary.

IMPACT OF STIGMA AND BIAS

Stigmatizing language and implicit bias toward patients with obesity significantly compromise the clinician–patient relationship and impede successful clinical treatment. Weight stigma and bias are detrimental to patient health, often leading to harmful responses, such as increased eating, depression, and failure to follow-up with healthcare providers (Puhl & Heuer, 2010). Unfortunately, weight stigma remains widespread, even among healthcare professionals. Studies show that weight discrimination has risen by 66% since 1995, paralleling the prevalence of racial discrimination (Andreyeva et al., 2008). It is crucial for healthcare professionals to examine their own assumptions and biases about patients with obesity, given the damaging impact these biases have on compassionate healthcare delivery. One useful tool for assessing personal implicit bias is Harvard University's Weight Implicit Association Test.

A vital aspect of patient-centered care is the use of inclusive, supportive language. Ivezaj and colleagues examined patient preferences regarding weight and eating-related terminology. Table 6.2 illustrates the proportion of participants who rated specific weight-related terms as either "very undesirable" or "very desirable" (Ivezaj et al., 2020).

Weight stigma and bias are pervasive throughout society and negatively impact both the physical and mental health of patients with obesity. This harmful behavior is not limited to the general public; healthcare professionals also exhibit bias toward patients with obesity. The rising prevalence of obesity has unveiled harmful stereotypes, which have led to behaviors that exacerbate the disease, such as binge eating and depression (Fruh, 2021).

Table 6.2 Proportions of Participants Rating Weight-Related Terms as "Very Undesirable" and "Very Desirable"

Very Undesirable N (%)	Term	Very Desirable N (%)
14 (12.3%)	Weight	16 (14%)
35 (30.7%)	Heaviness	2 (1.8%)
16 (14%)	BMI	16 (14%)
37 (32%)	Obesity	6 (5.3%)
22 (19.3)	Excess weight	7 (6.1%)
64 (56.1%	Fatness	1 (0.9)
43 (37.7%)	Excess weight	7 (6.1%)
45 (39.5%)	Large size	4 (3.5%)
17 (14.9)	Unhealthy body weight	9 (7.9%)
28 (24.6%)	Weight problem	11 (.6%)
22 (19.3%)	Unhealthy BMI	4 (3.5%)

Research shows that healthcare providers often spend less time with patients with obesity compared to those without, and patients with obesity are frequently labeled as non-compliant (Ginsburg et al., 2024). Unlike racial or gender biases, which are addressed by protective policies, similar safeguards for patients with obesity are lacking.

Several studies have documented that weight-based stigma from healthcare providers negatively affects patient care. A large-scale study involving more than 13,500 individuals across various countries found that among those who reported experiencing weight stigma, 66% encountered such behavior from healthcare providers (Fulton et al., 2023). Despite this, medical education still offers limited training on implicit bias and its impact on patient outcomes. It is essential for healthcare professionals to confront weight stigma while also expanding their understanding of the pathophysiology of obesity.

Implementing techniques to reduce bias in healthcare settings can improve both mental and physical health outcomes, ultimately leading to enhanced patient care. Healthcare professionals should avoid terms such as "fat" or "morbidly obese," which often trigger negative patient responses. Instead, they should use patient-first language, such as referring to someone as a "patient with obesity." Recognizing that a patient is more than their weight can foster more productive conversations about health and behaviors, resulting in improved patient experiences and outcomes. Healthcare environments should also be designed to ensure comfort and safety for patients with obesity. This includes providing appropriately sized chairs, larger gowns, discreetly placed scales, and larger blood pressure cuffs to meet the specific needs of patients.

Recognizing weight management as a sensitive topic, healthcare professionals should approach it thoughtfully, asking for permission before engaging in conversations about weight. Negative experiences related to weight management in healthcare settings can have adverse psychological consequences, leading to poor health behaviors and mental health challenges. Although weight may contribute to clinical conditions, simply advising a patient to "lose weight" is not a comprehensive solution to their overall health.

Raising awareness of obesity-related bias and discrimination should be an integral part of healthcare system training. Treating obesity like other complex chronic conditions will promote a more holistic treatment strategy that focuses on the whole patient, not just their eating habits. Implementing zero-tolerance policies for weight-based discrimination among healthcare professionals and their teams can help create a supportive and sensitive environment for all patients.

CONCLUSION

Empathetic and supportive communication, beginning the moment a patient enters the office and continuing throughout the care experience, is crucial for combating obesity bias in healthcare. Conducting clinical assessments in a compassionate, bias-free manner within a comfortable, accommodating environment is essential for achieving optimal health outcomes for patients with obesity. Recognizing the complexity of obesity and addressing stigma and bias, especially among healthcare providers, can pave the way for more productive patient–clinician relationships. The upcoming chapters will delve deeper into the detailed assessment and treatment plans that form the foundation of effective, patient-centered obesity care.

CLINICAL CONSIDERATIONS CHECKLIST: CULTURALLY TAILORED APPROACH TO OBESITY ASSESSMENT

This guide outlines key steps for engaging in a productive and compassionate clinical conversation with patients managing obesity. By following these motivational interviewing techniques, healthcare providers can foster a patient-centered approach that builds trust, addresses bias, and promotes sustainable health outcomes. It is essential to approach each conversation with sensitivity, actively addressing potential bias or stigma to create a safe and supportive environment for the patient.

Key Considerations in the Clinical Assessment

- *Patient History*: Medical, weight, family, psychological, and dietary history.
- *Physical Exam*: BMI, waist circumference, blood pressure, and signs of insulin resistance.

- *Lab Tests*: Fasting glucose, lipid panel, liver function, thyroid, and hormonal tests.
- *Comorbidities*: Cardiovascular risk, type 2 diabetes, and sleep apnea.
- *Behavioral/Psychological*: Assess for eating disorders, motivation, and mental health status.
- *Treatment Options*: Behavioral changes, pharmacotherapy, and surgery referrals.
- *Follow-Up and Monitoring*: Regular follow-up is crucial for monitoring treatment effectiveness, adjusting goals, and supporting the patient's progress.

Motivational Interviewing

Step	Action	Purpose
Step 1: Ask Permission	"Would it be okay if we discussed your weight today?"	Demonstrate compassion and develop trust in the clinician–provider relationship.
Step 2: Assess Understanding and History	"Do you know obesity is a complex medical disease? It is not your fault." "What has your experience been on your weight journey and with your health?"	Address implicit or explicit bias prior to the visit. Provide relevant information about obesity as a disease. Use active listening and empathy. Confirm the obesity classification using BMI and waist circumference. Establish disease severity with tools like the Edmonton Obesity Staging System.
Step 3: Advise on Management	"Obesity is a complex disease that needs individualized treatment. Let's discuss the best management for your unique health needs."	Review treatment options based on the patient's unique biological, psychological, and social factors. Create a personalized management plan.
Step 4: Agree on Goals	"Let's come up with personalized goals and an action plan that are sustainable for you."	Focus on practical, actionable goals that align with the patient's priorities. Emphasize sustainability in the action plan.
Step 5: Assist with Barriers	"Let's see what we can come up with to overcome this issue."	Promote a partnership with the patient by celebrating wins, discussing roadblocks, and generating solutions. Set goals for the next visit.

Section III

Opportunities

Fundamentals of Obesity Management Overview

Tiffani Bell-Washington, MD, MPH, MBA, FAPA, FOMA, DABOM, DABLM, Kathi Earles, MD, MPH, DABOM, and Sylvia Gonsahn-Bollie, MD, DABOM, FOMA

One of the most common misconceptions about body weight is that it is something that you should fully be able to control.

—Dr. Arya Sharma

Chapter 7 Highlights

- **Cultural Adaptation:** Culturally appropriate dietary plans and exercise programs that resonate with the patient's lived experience.
- **Behavioral Support:** Mental health support that addresses the role of systemic racism and social determinants of health in shaping psychological well-being.
- **Multidisciplinary Approach:** Effective care involves a coordinated team of medical, nutritional, and behavioral experts addressing all aspects of health.
- **Addressing Stigma:** Incorporate culturally sensitive mental health support to tackle stigma, stress, and systemic barriers impacting Black communities.
- **Long-Term Strategy:** Continuous support and follow-up are essential for preventing weight regain, making obesity management an ongoing partnership.

INTRODUCTION

Obesity is a multifaceted disease requiring a comprehensive approach to achieve sustainable weight loss and improve health outcomes. This chapter outlines key components of effective obesity management, offering healthcare professionals evidence-based strategies tailored to support Black patients in overcoming cultural, behavioral, and metabolic challenges. By understanding these principles, clinicians can develop more personalized

DOI: 10.1201/9781032622217-10

treatment plans that address the unique factors influencing obesity in Black communities. Details on pediatric obesity are covered in Chapter 13.

OVERVIEW: KEY COMPONENTS OF OBESITY MANAGEMENT

Obesity is a complex, chronic disease that involves biological, behavioral, and environmental factors. Successful treatment requires a multidisciplinary approach that includes medical professionals, registered dietitians, behavioral therapists, and exercise specialists. The focus must go beyond body mass index (BMI) and weight, and center on overall health, cardiometabolic improvement, and quality of life. This collaborative approach ensures that each aspect of a patient's health is addressed holistically, which is crucial for creating a sustainable path to overall well-being.

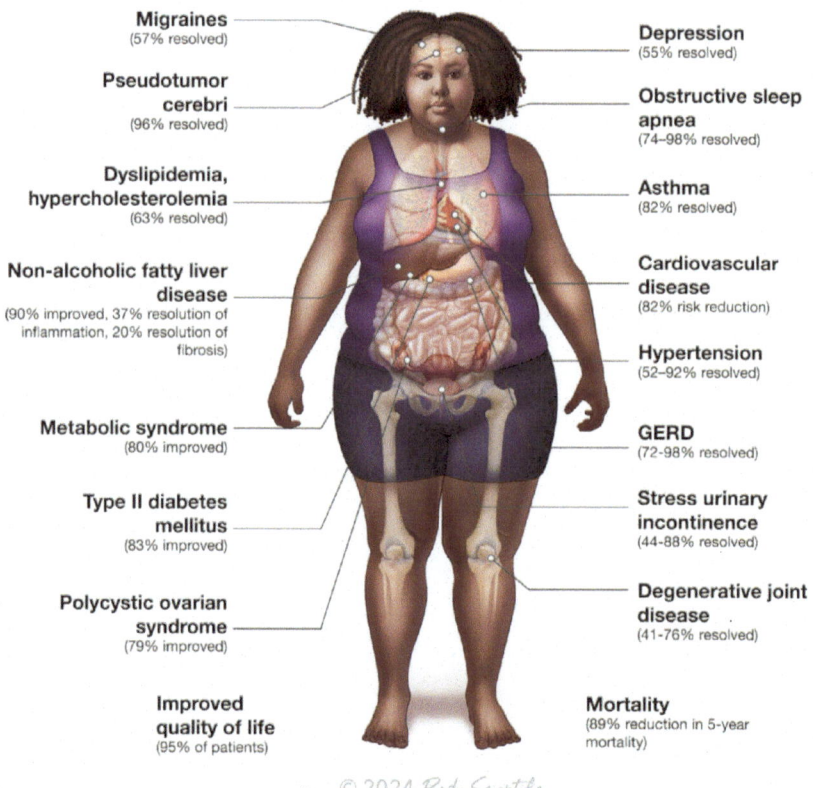

Improved Comorbidities post Bariatric Surgery

Migraines
(57% resolved)

Pseudotumor cerebri
(96% resolved)

Dyslipidemia, hypercholesterolemia
(63% resolved)

Non-alcoholic fatty liver disease
(90% improved, 37% resolution of inflammation, 20% resolution of fibrosis)

Metabolic syndrome
(80% improved)

Type II diabetes mellitus
(83% improved)

Polycystic ovarian syndrome
(79% improved)

Improved quality of life
(95% of patients)

Depression
(55% resolved)

Obstructive sleep apnea
(74–98% resolved)

Asthma
(82% resolved)

Cardiovascular disease
(82% risk reduction)

Hypertension
(52–92% resolved)

GERD
(72-98% resolved)

Stress urinary incontinence
(44-88% resolved)

Degenerative joint disease
(41-76% resolved)

Mortality
(89% reduction in 5-year mortality)

© 2024 Body Scientific

Referenece: https://asmbs.org/resources/metabolic-and-bariatric-surgery/

The essential components of effective obesity management include:

- **Lifestyle modifications,** such as dietary adjustments and increased physical activity (Chapter 8, Chapter 10).
- **Medical nutrition therapy (MNT)**, where a registered dietitian leads a personalized nutrition plan to optimize nutritional intake (Chapter 8).
- **Behavioral interventions and psychological support** to address emotional, cognitive, and mental health conditions (Chapter 9).
- **Pharmacotherapy** when appropriate (Chapter 11).
- **Bariatric and metabolic surgery** for eligible patients (Chapter 12).

A comprehensive, personalized treatment strategy typically involves a combination of these components. It is important for patients to understand that obesity is a lifelong condition that requires ongoing monitoring and adaptation of treatment plans. Long-term maintenance and follow-up are essential to prevent weight regain and sustain the health benefits achieved through obesity treatment.

This approach underscores that obesity is not a consequence of personal failure but a complex medical condition that demands individualized, empathetic care and continual support. Creating an unbiased and compassionate treatment environment is vital. As discussed in Chapter 5, individuals with higher body weight often avoid healthcare due to weight stigma, which is compounded by racial bias in Black communities. This leads to a lower likelihood of seeking healthcare, despite the availability of effective treatments. Social determinants of health, such as financial and social challenges and limited healthcare access, exacerbate the issue, as discussed in Chapter 4. An incorrect treatment approach can lead to severe health consequences, including disability and shortened lifespan (Washington et al., 2023).

ADDRESSING STIGMA AND ITS IMPACT ON CARE

Stigma associated with obesity is a well-documented barrier to healthcare, contributing to delayed medical care and poorer health outcomes. Black patients may face compounded stigma—not only from weight but also from racial discrimination in healthcare settings. This "double stigma" exacerbates barriers to seeking treatment, as highlighted in a study with Black adults suffering from behavioral health disorders (Yu et al., 2022). The study found that racial stigma and internalized self-stigma contributed to depressive symptoms, further hindering help-seeking behaviors.

DETAILS OF KEY COMPONENTS OF EFFECTIVE OBESITY MANAGEMENT

Lifestyle Modifications

Lifestyle changes form the cornerstone of obesity treatment. This includes a combination of dietary adjustments, physical activity, behavioral therapy, and ongoing support. Successful interventions should prioritize culturally relevant strategies that resonate with patients' lived experiences, dietary preferences, and socioeconomic contexts.

Medical Nutrition Therapy (MNT)

Personalized dietary interventions, guided by a registered dietitian or an obesity management specialist, are crucial for long-term weight management. Emphasis should be placed on reducing caloric intake, improving the nutritional quality of food, and ensuring dietary adequacy. For Black patients, this may involve incorporating culturally familiar foods and offering education on modifying traditional recipes for healthier outcomes.

Physical Activity and Exercise Prescription

Regular physical activity is critical for both weight loss and maintenance. Exercise recommendations should be tailored to the patient's preferences, fitness levels, comorbidities, and social determinants of health, such as neighborhood conditions. Culturally relevant activities—such as community sports, dance, or family-based physical activity—can enhance patient engagement and adherence.

Behavioral Interventions and Psychological Support

Addressing the psychological aspects of obesity is essential. This includes body image, self-esteem, and stress management. Motivational interviewing, goal-setting, cognitive-behavioral therapy, and mindfulness practices can help patients sustain healthier behaviors. In Black patients, it is particularly important to consider the impact of systemic racism and social determinants of health on mental well-being.

Pharmacotherapy

In addition to lifestyle changes, pharmacotherapy may be appropriate for patients with a BMI ≥27 kg/m² with weight-related conditions such as diabetes, hypertension, or sleep apnea, or a BMI ≥30 kg/m². Selecting the right medication requires careful evaluation of the patient's overall health, comorbid conditions, and potential side effects. Shared decision-making, which respects patient preferences and social circumstances, is critical for treatment adherence.

Bariatric and Metabolic Surgery

Bariatric surgery is an option for individuals with metabolic disease and a BMI of 30–34.9 kg/m² or a BMI of 35 kg/m² or higher, regardless of the presence of obesity-related conditions. Comprehensive pre- and post-surgical care, including nutritional counseling, mental health support, and long-term follow-up, is essential to optimize outcomes. For Black patients, it is important to consider the unique risks and benefits while emphasizing equitable access to these procedures.

Long-Term Maintenance and Follow-Up

Obesity is a chronic condition requiring ongoing management. It is important to set expectations for long-term treatment from the outset to prevent disappointment from weight regain, which is common when treatment is not sustained. Regular follow-ups, at least every 6 months, and continuous support are key to preventing weight regain and maintaining cardiometabolic benefits. This phase may include in-office visits, remote monitoring, telehealth check-ins, group support, and addressing new barriers as they arise.

KEY COMPONENTS OF OBESITY MANAGEMENT QUICK LIST

Component	Description	Key Considerations
Lifestyle Modifications	Dietary changes, physical activity, and behavioral interventions	Focus on culturally relevant strategies and support.
Medical Nutrition Therapy	Structured dietary guidance for weight management	Tailor to cultural preferences and traditional diets.
Physical Activity	Regular exercise for weight loss and maintenance	Encourage community engagement and accessibility.
Behavioral Interventions	Psychological support, goal-setting, and stress management	Address systemic stressors and support mental health.
Pharmacotherapy	Medications to support weight loss in addition to lifestyle changes	Individualized selection based on comorbidities.

(Continued)

(Continued)

Component	Description	Key Considerations
Bariatric and Metabolic Surgery	Surgical interventions for severe obesity	Ensure equitable access and comprehensive care.
Long-Term Maintenance	Ongoing support to prevent weight regain	Emphasize regular follow-ups and patient-centered care.

CONCLUSION

In managing obesity, a personalized, culturally informed approach is critical for ensuring sustainable health outcomes. This chapter has outlined the key components of an effective obesity management strategy, from lifestyle modifications and Medical Nutrition Therapy to behavioral interventions and pharmacotherapy. Each of these treatment elements is crucial and will be explored in detail in the following chapters. By addressing the unique cultural, behavioral, and medical challenges that Black patients face, healthcare professionals can provide more effective, compassionate care. Ultimately, a multidisciplinary approach, combined with long-term support, is essential for achieving lasting success in obesity management.

CLINICAL CONSIDERATIONS CHECKLIST: FUNDAMENTALS OF OBESITY MANAGEMENT

1. Patient Assessment
   - Take comprehensive medical, dietary, and physical activity history.
   - Screen for comorbid conditions (e.g., hypertension, diabetes).
   - Assess for psychological factors impacting weight management.
   - Evaluate previous weight loss attempts and barriers.
   - *Pre-Appointment Questionnaire:* Include the following questions:
     1. What is your primary reason for seeking obesity treatment?
     2. Have you previously tried to lose weight? If yes, what strategies have you used?
     3. How would you describe your current eating habits?
     4. What barriers do you currently face that make weight management challenging?
     5. How do you feel about your current level of physical activity?
     6. On a scale of 1–10, how motivated are you to make lifestyle changes?
     7. What are your biggest stressors, and how do they impact your health?
     8. Have you been diagnosed with any conditions that may impact your weight?

9. What does success look like to you in terms of weight management?
10. Is there anything else your healthcare provider should know?

2. Individualized Treatment Planning
- Set realistic weight loss goals collaboratively.
- Consider cultural, social, and economic factors.
- Develop a stepwise treatment plan incorporating dietary, physical activity, and behavioral strategies.

3. Behavioral and Psychological Support
- Implement motivational interviewing and cognitive-behavioral therapy.
- Address emotional eating, body image, and stressors.
- Support overcoming weight bias and stigma.

4. Pharmacotherapy Considerations
- Determine candidacy for anti-obesity medications.
- Discuss risks, benefits, and expectations with the patient.
- Monitor for efficacy and potential side effects.

5. Surgical Evaluation
- Assess eligibility for metabolic and bariatric surgery.
- Provide thorough pre-operative counseling and education.
- Plan for long-term nutritional and psychological follow-up.

6. Long-Term Maintenance Strategy
- Schedule regular follow-up appointments.
- Provide resources for ongoing support (e.g., support groups, telehealth).
- Reassess and adjust the plan as needed to maintain progress.

Chapter 8

Nutrition and Lifestyle Intervention and Inclusive Obesity Care

Daphne Bryan, MD, DABOM,
Tiffani Bell-Washington, MD, MPH, MBA, FAPA,
FOMA, DABOM, DABLM, and
Sylvia Gonsahn-Bollie, MD, DABOM, FOMA

> We need to focus on a national effort to reverse the trend of obesity by educating people on how to choose nutritious foods, increase physical activity, and manage stress, with the ultimate goal of achieving optimal health for all Americans at every stage of life.
>
> —Dr. Regina Benjamin, MD, 18th U.S. Surgeon General

Chapter 8 Highlights

- Comprehensive obesity care should prioritize sustainable, personalized treatment plans, including dietary changes, exercise, and behavioral support tailored to individual and cultural preferences.
- Social determinants of health (SDOH), such as economic stability and access to healthy food, play a critical role in obesity rates, particularly in African American communities. Addressing SDOH is essential for effective nutrition and lifestyle interventions.
- Malnutrition is a concern in people with obesity. Eating plans must address nutrient gaps while promoting healthy weight and overall health.

INTRODUCTION

Nutrition and lifestyle changes are essential components of effective obesity care, directly influencing health outcomes and long-term weight management. Nutrition refers to the process of obtaining the food necessary for health and growth, while lifestyle changes encompass modifications to daily habits, such as physical activity, sleep patterns, reducing substance use, fostering community support, and managing stress. Both optimal nutrition and healthy lifestyle habits are key to addressing obesity.

DOI: 10.1201/9781032622217-11

It is equally important to consider personal preferences, which are often shaped by culture and community. In the Black community, individualized approaches to care are especially critical, as conventional nutrition guidelines and resources have historically failed to incorporate cultural preferences. While many cultural practices offer health benefits, some traditions or habits may present challenges, particularly in communities affected by social determinants of health (SDOH) that limit access to healthy foods, safe environments, and quality healthcare.

The goal of nutrition and lifestyle interventions should be to honor the positive aspects of cultural identity while supporting improvements in eating patterns and daily habits. This chapter will explore the following key topics:

- The importance of personalized nutrition and lifestyle interventions in obesity care
- How lifestyle medicine supports weight management and reduces health disparities in Black populations
- Nutritional status and food security
- The effectiveness of various eating plans for weight loss
- The impact of social determinants of health on nutrition and weight management
- The relationship between trauma and obesity
- The role of behavioral support in long-term weight management success
- The significance of community and social support in improving health outcomes for Black populations

IMPORTANCE OF PERSONALIZED NUTRITION AND LIFESTYLE INTERVENTIONS IN OBESITY CARE

Lifestyle medicine is a medical approach that uses evidence-based lifestyle changes, such as good nutrition, physical activity, sleep, stress management, social connection, and avoiding harmful substances, to prevent, treat, and often reverse chronic diseases (American College of Lifestyle Medicine, 2024). Scientific evidence confirms that lifestyle changes can be beneficial in obesity treatment by supporting both weight loss and improving health outcomes (Look AHEAD Research Group et al., 2007, 2013). The goal of obesity treatment should extend beyond reaching a specific number on the scale. Obesity is associated with more than 200 diseases that affect every organ in the body. Therefore, comprehensive obesity care aims to prevent or improve complications of obesity such as diabetes, cardiovascular disease, and orthopedic conditions that lead to joint replacement or disability, and organ damage or failure.

Although there have been revolutionary advances in obesity medications and bariatric surgery in the past two decades, lifestyle medicine and personalized lifestyle modifications remain foundational to obesity treatment. In Black populations, where systemic barriers and health inequities have historically limited access to health, lifestyle modification can be a helpful step in management (Rippe, 2018). By addressing not only diet and physical activity, but also sleep, stress management, and social support, lifestyle medicine can provide a holistic framework for sustainable health.

Multiple large, multicenter trials, such as the Diabetes Prevention Program (DPP) and Look AHEAD (Action for Health in Diabetes), have shown that lifestyle modifications resulting in at least 7% weight loss are associated with better glucose control and reduced use of antihypertensives, statins, and insulin (Look AHEAD Research Group et al., 2007, 2013). Additionally, these lifestyle changes improve conditions like sleep apnea, fatty liver disease, and kidney disease (Foster et al., 2009; Kuna et al., 2013). At 10% weight loss, there is a reduced risk of fatal and nonfatal cardiovascular events (Rubino et al., 2023). It is important to note that in cardiovascular patients who have systolic or diastolic heart failure, there is a paradoxical increase in mortality with weight reduction (Hamzeh et al., 2017), further emphasizing the importance of individualized, comprehensive treatment planning that extends beyond weight loss alone.

Lifestyle changes encompass movement, eating habits, sleep, and stress management. The process begins with educating patients, especially about what constitutes a healthy eating pattern. Evidence suggests that focusing on reducing calories consumed versus calories burned leads to greater success in weight reduction (Garvey et al., 2016). Keeping a food diary, either paper or electronic, is crucial for individuals who do not eat the same thing each day. Daily repetition of meals is unsustainable, and maintaining a food diary can be challenging for many. Therefore, using available apps and taking photos of food can be helpful. The photographed food can be used as a memory cue to log entries into the food diary when time permits. A food diary offers a realistic view of daily food intake, reduces mindless eating, and can help patients make mindful choices.

For Black people, lifestyle medicine not only supports sustainable weight loss but also helps reduce the risk of comorbidities such as diabetes, hypertension, and cardiovascular disease, which occur at higher rates in this population (American College of Lifestyle Medicine, 2021). By integrating cultural dietary preferences, incorporating enjoyable physical activities, and addressing stressors unique to the Black community—such as racism and socioeconomic barriers—lifestyle medicine can offer a powerful, personalized approach that respects cultural identity and promotes long-term health.

Key Elements of Lifestyle Medicine in Black Populations

- **Nutrition:** Creating culturally tailored eating plans that incorporate traditional foods and recipes while maintaining a focus on nutrient density and balanced macronutrient intake (Rippe, 2018).
- **Physical Activity:** Encouraging forms of movement that are culturally relevant and accessible, such as dance, group exercise, or community walking programs (American College of Lifestyle Medicine, 2021).
- **Stress Management:** Incorporating mindfulness practices, such as prayer, meditation, and yoga, which have been shown to reduce stress and promote emotional well-being, especially in communities of color (Randall et al., 2015).
- **Sleep:** Addressing sleep hygiene and its impact on weight and overall health. Screen for sleep disorders given the higher prevalence of sleep conditions in Black communities (Grandner et al., 2016; Johnson et al., 2019).
- **Community Support:** Building a network of support that includes family, friends, and healthcare professionals to reinforce positive lifestyle changes and address challenges like time constraints, food insecurity, or limited exercise opportunities (Assari, 2018; Holt et al., 2014).

NUTRITIONAL STATUS AND FOOD SECURITY IN PEOPLE WITH OBESITY

When discussing nutrition and obesity, the conversation often shifts to dieting and weight loss; however, nutrition encompasses much more. Nutrition is the "food or nourishment" the body needs and, in a disciplinary sense, "the study of nutrients in food, how the body uses them, and the relationship between diet, health, and disease" (Hickson et al., 2024). A comprehensive approach to obesity care should prioritize nutrient-dense food options to address both weight management and overall health status. We must emphasize the importance of not just weight loss but also focus on improving dietary quality and food diversity as key components of obesity treatment (Johnson et al., 2022). Limiting the discussion of nutrition in obesity care solely to food restriction and weight loss misses the opportunity to optimize the nutritional status and overall health of individuals with obesity.

Furthermore, people with obesity are at risk of malnutrition due to several factors, including chronic inflammation from excess adipose tissue, an altered gut microbiome that favors unhealthy bacteria, and the consumption of low-nutrient foods. Research has shown that people with obesity often have low levels of essential vitamins such as B1, B6, B12, C, and D, as well as minerals like iron and zinc (Kobylińska et al., 2022). This risk is heightened by food insecurity, disproportionately affecting African Americans due to systemic barriers such as socioeconomic status. Many Black communities face challenges in accessing nutrient-rich foods, leading to both malnutrition and obesity (Eskandari et al., 2022; Johnson et al., 2022).

In some cases, food insecurity, defined as the lack of sufficient food to meet one's needs, contributes to poor health outcomes, including obesity. For example, a study of Black women in an urban U.S. city found that food insecurity exacerbated obesity and related health conditions (Vedovato et al., 2016). Linked to food insecurity is the issue of food deserts—areas with limited access to supermarkets or outlets selling nutrient-dense foods. A study of more than 97,000 California residents showed that food deserts in high-poverty, predominantly Black neighborhoods are associated with higher rates of overweight and obesity, whereas low-poverty food deserts do not show the same association. However, other research, such as a larger study using National Health Interview Survey data, found that food insecurity was not always associated with overweight/obesity in Black men and women (Hernandez et al., 2017). These conflicting findings highlight the variability within Black communities, demonstrating that a one-size-fits-all approach to nutrition and obesity care will not work.

These insights reveal that, while dietary modification is a critical component of obesity treatment, a comprehensive approach to nutrition must assess dietary quality, diversity, and food access. Clinicians should be aware of food assistance programs in their communities and advocate for those that prioritize healthful, nutrient-rich foods. With a growing movement toward providing healthier food options through these programs, the opportunity to improve both malnutrition and obesity outcomes is becoming more accessible.

Addressing malnutrition in people with obesity requires not only improving nutrient intake but also selecting eating plans that provide balanced macronutrients and are sustainable in the long term, tailored to individual health needs and preferences. The next two sections will explore various eating plans and considerations for individualizing these plans.

MACRONUTRIENT COMPOSITION AND INDIVIDUALIZATION

There is mixed evidence on which diet process or macronutrient composition is most effective for weight loss, likely because no two people are alike. Excess calories and a sedentary lifestyle generally result in weight gain, but the type of fat (trans vs. unsaturated) and carbohydrate (simple vs. complex) consumed also plays a role. Research on the Mediterranean diet, DASH diet, and other trials comparing macronutrient-based plans has not identified a consistent "winner" in terms of weight loss. Success seems to be tied to calorie deficits, low sugar intake, inclusion of vegetables and lean protein, and cultural and financial considerations (Shai et al., 2008; Hall & Guo, 2017).

TYPES OF EATING PLANS

Despite extensive research and clinical experience in treating obesity, there remains no single eating plan proven to be universally superior for weight loss, weight maintenance, and optimizing health (Johnston et al., 2014). This is largely because every individual has unique dietary needs and preferences. Therefore, when selecting an eating plan, it's essential to consider personal preferences, health conditions, food access, and the ability to maintain the plan long term.

Eating plans can either focus on a balanced-calorie approach or target specific macronutrient distributions, such as fats, carbohydrates (CHO), and proteins.

Low-Calorie Diets

Low-calorie diets (900–1100 calories per day) and very-low-calorie diets (800–900 calories per day) can be achieved using portion-controlled products like meal replacements, frozen foods, or prepackaged meals. These options ease the burden of daily meal prep, which can feel overwhelming for individuals beginning lifestyle changes for weight management (Garvey et al., 2016). Low-calorie plans also include the Mediterranean and DASH (Dietary Approach to Stop Hypertension) diets. Although not specifically weight loss focused, these diets often result in weight reduction. The Mediterranean diet is associated with cardiovascular risk reduction and diabetes prevention, while the DASH diet was created to lower blood pressure. Combined with exercise, the DASH diet can also support weight loss (Shai et al., 2008; Yancy et al., 2004). Both are considered balanced-calorie eating plans and do not emphasize specific macronutrient counts.

Low-Fat Diets

Low-fat diets are designed to improve cardiovascular health and support weight loss, although they have not been proven to be more effective than low-carbohydrate diets (Hall & Guo, 2017). These diets typically limit fat to less than 30% of total energy intake or approximately 30 grams per 1,000 kcal. However, when low-fat diets became popular, there was a tendency to increase carbohydrate intake, which some argue contributed to the obesity epidemic. An effective low-fat eating plan should limit saturated fats and simple carbohydrates, while incorporating complex carbohydrates such as vegetables (Shan et al., 2020).

Low-Carbohydrate Diets

Low-carbohydrate diets limit carbohydrate intake to 60–130 grams per day and emphasize healthy fats, such as monounsaturated and polyunsaturated fats. Very-low-carb diets restrict carbohydrate intake to less than 60 grams per day. These plans exclude sugary foods, beverages, and calorie-dense snacks. One significant benefit of low-carb diets is their ability to increase HDL cholesterol and lower triglycerides. However, very-low-carb diets, such as the Atkins diet, are often associated with side effects such as constipation, headaches, halitosis, and muscle cramps (Fung et al., 2010).

High-Protein Diets

High-protein diets, in which at least 20% of daily calories come from protein, typically include lean meat or vegetable-based protein. These diets promote satiety, increase thermogenesis, and can be beneficial for weight management. Furthermore, eating plans that are high in plant protein and unsaturated fats have been linked to lower mortality risks compared to low-carbohydrate, high-saturated fat diets (Gardner et al., 2018).

Intermittent Fasting

Intermittent fasting, a popular eating approach, may be used independently or complement any eating meal plan. Intermittent fasting limits calorie intake by restricting the time during which patients eat. This can be done by limiting eating to an 8- to 10-hour window or alternating fasting days with regular eating days. These plans are difficult to sustain, and neither have consistently shown significant weight loss or cardiovascular improvements beyond regular calorie-restriction eating plans (De Souza et al., 2021).

Mediterranean Diet

The Mediterranean diet has been shown to have many health benefits, particularly for heart health and inflammatory conditions. It is a plant-based eating pattern that emphasizes fruits, vegetables, whole grains, healthy fats like olive oil, and lean proteins such as fish and poultry (Martínez-González et al., 2019). However, for people who did not grow up with a Mediterranean eating plan, trying to eat this way can feel culturally limiting. Fortunately, foods from the African Diaspora can be incorporated into a culturally specific Mediterranean eating plan, offering familiar flavors and ingredients while maintaining the diet's health benefits. For example, dishes like black-eyed peas or pigeon peas can provide excellent plant-based protein sources, while okra and collard greens offer nutrient-dense vegetables. Staple grains like rice can be replaced with whole grains like quinoa or bulgur, and heart-healthy fats from foods like plantains, ackee, or groundnuts (peanuts) align with the Mediterranean focus on healthy fats. Seasoning dishes with herbs and spices common in African, Caribbean, or Southern cuisine, such as cumin, ginger, and turmeric, can make meals both comforting and flavorful. This approach allows individuals to enjoy the benefits of the Mediterranean diet while honoring their cultural food heritage.

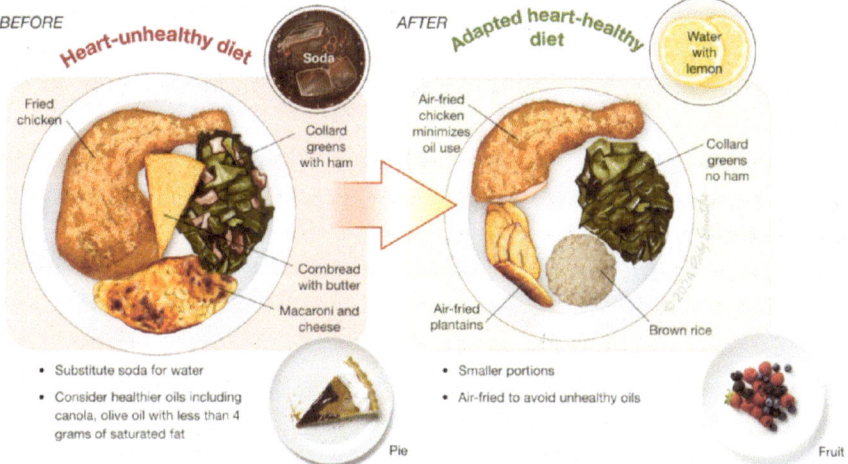

Regardless of the eating plan chosen, it is important to ensure that all macronutrients—healthy fats, complex carbohydrates, and lean or plant-based protein—are incorporated. Micronutrients like vitamins, minerals, and gut-friendly foods containing prebiotics and probiotics should also be consumed regularly to promote overall health. Cultural preferences and individual circumstances should guide the personalization of each plan to improve long-term adherence and sustainability.

CONSULTATION AND PERSONALIZATION

It is highly recommended to include individual consultations with a registered dietitian when creating a personalized eating plan. The best outcomes are linked to patients who participate in selecting and creating their eating plans. Cost, cultural influences, personal preferences, and health conditions should all be considered when designing a plan. For instance, patients with kidney disease should avoid high-protein eating plans. To ensure sustainability, it is important to incorporate foods that are common to the patient's culture, such as substituting brown rice for White rice or baked pork chops for fried ones, all while staying within calorie, fat, and sugar limits (Garvey et al., 2016).

BEHAVIORAL SUPPORT

Behavioral support plays a key role in long-term weight loss success. There is a known connection between childhood trauma, including physical, mental, or sexual abuse, neglect, or food insecurity, and adult obesity. The exact mechanism is unclear, but early trauma may lead to self-soothing with food. More research is needed to fully understand the connection between trauma and obesity (Wiss & Brewerton, 2020). In Chapter 9, the behavioral aspects of obesity care will be discussed in more detail.

ROLE OF RACISM AND SOCIAL DETERMINANTS OF HEALTH

Limited access to affordable, healthy food is a significant consequence of racism's impact on the social determinants of health across the African Diaspora. Systemic racism restricts access to nutritious food in low-income, predominantly African-descended populations in the United States, Caribbean, South America, and Europe. As a result, these communities often rely on processed, high-calorie foods, which increases the risk of obesity. Social determinants like economic stability, education quality, and neighborhood safety—discussed in Chapter 4—are all negatively affected by systemic racism. In these underserved areas, cultural traditions also adapt to the limited availability of ingredients, further contributing to poor nutrition and obesity (Eskandari et al., 2022; Hernandez et al., 2017). However, community-based programs are working to break this cycle by improving access to healthy food and empowering residents. U.S.-based organizations such as Roots for Life, the Center for Black Health & Equity, and Feeding America are tackling food insecurity through education, local initiatives, and food distribution networks aimed at strengthening food security and nutrition in Black communities. These grassroots efforts highlight the power of the community to create healthier futures despite systemic challenges.

CONCLUSION

A comprehensive and personalized approach to obesity care is essential. Nutrition and lifestyle interventions should not focus solely on weight loss but should also address malnutrition, social determinants of health, and individual preferences to promote overall health and well-being. Sustainable weight management is best achieved through tailored eating plans, behavioral support, and an understanding of the broader social factors that influence health outcomes. Marginalized communities, such as Black and low-income populations who often face food insecurity, limited access to healthy foods, and systemic barriers like racism, should be a priority. By integrating these components, clinicians can help patients achieve long-term success in both health and weight management.

CLINICAL CONSIDERATIONS CHECKLIST: NUTRITION AND LIFESTYLE FACTORS

The following checklist is created to facilitate a holistic and individualized conversation between the clinician and the patient, ensuring that nutrition, lifestyle, and social factors are all addressed during the visit. Patients are encouraged to complete the checklist before the visit so the clinician can review it ahead of time.

- What are your current eating habits and food preferences? Are there any foods from your culture that are "essential" to you?

- How do your current sleep and stress levels impact your eating and physical activity?

- Have you experienced any challenges accessing healthy foods? If so, please explain.

- How do you currently manage your weight, and what past approaches have worked or not worked for you?

- Are there any specific health conditions (e.g., diabetes, cardiovascular disease) that impact your dietary needs?

- How much time and energy can you realistically dedicate to meal planning, preparation, and exercise?

- What is your experience with tracking food intake, such as keeping a food diary or using apps?

- How do your current sleep and stress levels impact your eating and physical activity?

Chapter 9

Behavioral Impact and Interventions in the Treatment of Obesity

Tiffani Bell-Washington, MD, MPH, MBA, FAPA, FOMA, DABOM, DABLM, Sylvia Gonsahn-Bollie, MD, DABOM, FOMA, and Sharon Dodd, MD

> Emotional well-being is more than the absence of a mental illness. It's that resource within each of us which allows us to reach ever closer to our full potential, and which also enables us to be resilient in the face of adversity.
>
> —Dr. Vivek Murthy, 19th U.S. Surgeon General

Chapter 9 Highlights

- **Cultural Stigma and Mental Health in Obesity:** Addressing cultural stigma, trauma, and mental health conditions through a culturally sensitive approach is crucial for effective obesity management in the Black community.
- **Behavioral Therapies Tailored for Readiness to Change:** Adapting interventions such as motivational interviewing and culturally adapted CBT using the Stages of Change model can improve patient engagement and outcomes.
- **Impact of Psychiatric Medications on Weight:** Selecting weight-neutral or weight-reducing psychiatric medications, such as SSRIs or GLP-1 receptor agonists, can minimize weight gain while supporting mental health.

INTRODUCTION

The intersection of mental health and obesity is a complex and bidirectional relationship that significantly impacts overall health outcomes. Research has shown that individuals with obesity are at a higher risk for developing mental health disorders, such as depression, anxiety, and binge eating disorder,

DOI: 10.1201/9781032622217-12

due to a variety of factors including societal stigma, discrimination, and low self-esteem: This increased risk of mental health disorders is consistent in both adults and children with obesity and independent of other risk factors (Lindberg et al., 2020). This chapter examines the complicated interaction between mental health and obesity that is frequently ignored and amplifies culturally tailored solutions.

DOUBLE STIGMA: OBESITY AND MENTAL HEALTH

Stigma, as defined by Merriam-Webster's dictionary, is a set of negative and unfair beliefs that a society or group of people have about something. In the Black community, mental health issues may be seen as taboo. Non-treatment of mental health issues leads to worse outcomes for patients. Obesity and mental health stigma are two of the most widely accepted forms of stigma and bias. Research supports that Black culture is more accepting of larger and curvier body types, which may lead to more satisfaction with body image, even if one technically has obesity or overweight (Spinner, 2022). On the other hand, by focusing on the impact of weight on daily functioning, health consequences, and quality of life, Black people can increase participation in weight loss programs that are culturally sensitive and community based (Alick et al., 2023).

The psychological distress associated with weight stigma can exacerbate unhealthy eating patterns, reduce motivation for physical activity, and contribute to emotional eating, creating a vicious cycle that perpetuates both obesity and poor mental health. Moreover, the neurobiological mechanisms underlying these conditions, such as dysregulation of the hypothalamic–pituitary–adrenal (HPA) axis and altered neurotransmitter pathways, further complicate the relationship, making it difficult to treat one condition without addressing the other (Mikulska et al., 2021).

Comprehensive care models that incorporate mental health support, nutritional counseling, and behavioral strategies are essential for breaking the cycle between obesity and mental health challenges, ultimately improving the quality of life for affected individuals.

UNDERSTANDING BEHAVIORAL THERAPY IN THE BLACK COMMUNITY

Behavioral therapy is a structured approach that utilizes psychological techniques to promote long-term behavior change. This intervention is fundamental in managing obesity, as it addresses the mental and emotional barriers to healthy lifestyle changes. Given the complex interplay of cultural, social, and environmental factors influencing obesity in the Black community, behavioral interventions must be adapted to meet these unique needs (Tremblay et al., 2017). The Black community faces unique stressors such as systemic racism, socioeconomic inequalities, and cultural stigma, which is not adequately addressed in standard weight management programs (Hargreaves et al., 2020). Therefore, behavioral therapies must integrate a culturally sensitive approach and consider the social determinants of health that disproportionately impact Black individuals.

MULTIDISCIPLINARY TEAM APPROACH: INTEGRATING LIFESTYLE MEDICINE AND PSYCHIATRY

A successful obesity treatment plan in the Black community requires a comprehensive, multidisciplinary approach that integrates lifestyle medicine, lifestyle psychiatry, and community support. Lifestyle medicine emphasizes the use of evidence-based therapeutic lifestyle changes such as improved diet, regular physical activity, adequate sleep, stress management, and social connection to prevent and treat chronic diseases (Lianov, 2023). In parallel, lifestyle psychiatry incorporates similar principles but focuses on using these strategies to prevent and treat mental health disorders. Both approaches are essential in a holistic treatment plan for obesity in the Black community, where physical and mental health are closely intertwined (Earles et al., 2020). Specifically, lifestyle medicine and psychiatry may include psychological support and behavioral therapy, nutrition counseling, and health counseling.

Psychological Support and Behavioral Therapy

Psychological support is a critical component in managing obesity, particularly in addressing underlying mental health conditions such as depression, anxiety, and trauma, which are prevalent among Black individuals. Behavioral strategies such as cognitive-behavioral therapy (CBT), dialectical behavior therapy (DBT), and acceptance and commitment therapy (ACT) are effective in reducing emotional eating, improving self-esteem, and managing stress (Nogueira et al., 2023). Culturally adapted CBT and mindfulness-based stress reduction (MBSR) programs have shown promise in reducing binge eating and emotional dysregulation in African American women (Goode et al., 2022). Including stress management techniques that incorporate the patient's cultural and spiritual beliefs, such as prayer and community support, can enhance adherence and improve outcomes.

Nutrition Counseling with a Cultural Lens

Nutritional counseling tailored to the Black community must go beyond conventional dietary recommendations by incorporating cultural preferences and socioeconomic factors (Babatunde et al., 2020). For example, incorporating traditional African American dishes prepared in healthier ways respects cultural heritage while promoting nutritional changes. Programs like the DASH diet (Dietary Approaches to Stop Hypertension), which includes traditional foods like collard greens and sweet potatoes, have shown efficacy in reducing hypertension and improving weight management in African Americans (Earles et al., 2020). Furthermore, addressing food deserts, access to affordable healthy foods, and the impact of advertising unhealthy foods in low-income Black neighborhoods is crucial for sustainable dietary changes (Cooksey Stowers et al., 2020).

Health Coaching: Bridging Knowledge and Action

Health coaching is essential in bridging the gap between knowledge and behavior change, providing ongoing support, accountability, and motivation. In the Black community, health coaches who share the cultural background of their clients are more likely to establish trust and promote long-term engagement (Joo & Liu, 2021). Health coaching techniques such as motivational interviewing and personalized goal setting can help patients overcome barriers related to stress, environmental constraints, and socioeconomic disparities (Earles et al., 2020).

STRESS

Chronic stress is a well-documented contributor to both mental health disorders and obesity, serving as a significant factor in the development and persistence of both conditions. Prolonged stress activates the hypothalamic–pituitary–adrenal (HPA) axis, leading to elevated levels of cortisol, a stress hormone that promotes fat storage and increased appetite, particularly for high-calorie, sugary foods. During the COVID-19 pandemic, stress levels were notably elevated, causing many individuals to adopt maladaptive coping mechanisms such as emotional eating and reduced physical activity, thereby worsening obesity and mental health outcomes (Melamed et al., 2022). Addressing stress through behavioral therapies such as mindfulness-based stress reduction (MBSR) or cognitive-behavioral therapy (CBT) can play a crucial role in breaking the cycle between stress, overeating, and weight gain.

TRAUMA AND ADVERSE CHILDHOOD EXPERIENCES (ACEs)

Trauma, particularly adverse childhood experiences (ACEs), has been strongly linked to both obesity and mental health conditions (Mahmood et al., 2023). ACEs include experiences such as abuse, neglect, or household dysfunction, which disrupt normal development and increase the risk of obesity and psychiatric disorders in adulthood. Studies show that individuals with high ACE scores are more likely to engage in unhealthy behaviors such as emotional eating and substance use, both of which contribute to obesity and worsen mental health (Zielińska et al., 2024). Trauma-informed care, which emphasizes safety, trust, and empowerment, is essential in addressing these issues. Integrating trauma-sensitive approaches in obesity treatment can improve patient outcomes by reducing the psychological burden that perpetuates disordered eating and weight gain.

MENTAL HEALTH CONDITIONS

The relationship between mental health disorders and obesity is bidirectional and complex. Conditions such as depression, anxiety, and post-traumatic stress disorder (PTSD) are commonly seen in individuals with obesity. Depression, for instance, is associated with increased appetite and weight gain due to altered serotonin pathways and the adoption of sedentary behaviors. Conversely, people with obesity are more prone to developing depression and anxiety due to social stigma and low self-esteem (Blasco et al., 2020; Leutner et al., 2023). Addressing mental health as part of obesity management requires a comprehensive approach that includes screening for psychiatric symptoms and providing appropriate psychological interventions.

EATING DISORDERS AND DISORDERED EATING

Disordered eating patterns, such as binge eating, night eating syndrome, and food addiction, are prevalent in individuals with obesity and are often exacerbated by co-occurring mental health conditions. Binge eating disorder (BED), in particular, is characterized by recurrent episodes of consuming large amounts of food in a short period, accompanied by feelings of loss of control and distress. During the COVID-19 pandemic, the prevalence of disordered eating behaviors increased due to elevated stress and anxiety levels (Melamed et al., 2022). Interventions such as cognitive-behavioral therapy (CBT) and dialectical behavior therapy (DBT) have been found to be effective in treating BED and other forms of disordered eating by addressing both emotional regulation and problematic eating patterns.

PSYCHIATRIC MEDICATIONS AND WEIGHT MANAGEMENT: IMPLICATIONS FOR BLACK PATIENTS

The intersection of psychiatric medications and obesity management is particularly relevant in the Black community, given the high prevalence of both obesity and mental health conditions. Many psychiatric medications, particularly antipsychotics and certain mood stabilizers, are associated with significant weight gain, which can exacerbate obesity and increase the risk of metabolic disorders (McIntyre et al., 2024). Additionally, some antidepressants and mood stabilizers have weight-neutral or weight-reducing effects, making them more suitable options for patients struggling with obesity and psychiatric comorbidities (Shrivastava & Johnston, 2010). The following sections explore the distinctions between weight-inducing, weight-neutral, and weight-reducing medications in the context of obesity and mental health management.

Weight-Inducing Medications

Antipsychotic medications, such as olanzapine and risperidone, have been shown to significantly increase weight due to their effects on appetite regulation and metabolic pathways (McIntyre et al., 2024). These medications may disproportionately impact Black individuals due to genetic and metabolic differences, as well as barriers to accessing weight management support services (Saunders et al., 2016). This makes it imperative for clinicians to conduct regular metabolic monitoring and consider switching to weight-neutral medications when clinically appropriate (Earles et al., 2020).

Weight-Neutral and Weight-Reducing Medications

SSRIs and other antidepressants are generally considered weight-neutral, although individual responses vary (Shrivastava & Johnston, 2010). Recent research has highlighted the benefits of GLP-1 receptor agonists, which not only promote weight loss but also show promise in improving mood and reducing emotional eating (Earles et al., 2020). These medications may be particularly beneficial for Black patients, who have higher rates of obesity-related comorbidities and may struggle with weight gain from other psychiatric treatments.

CULTIVATING READINESS FOR CHANGE IN THE BLACK COMMUNITY

Assessing readiness for change is crucial when working with Black patients who may have varying levels of motivation and awareness regarding obesity-related health risks (Prochaska & DiClemente, 1983). The Transtheoretical

Model of Change (TTM) helps clinicians tailor interventions based on the patient's stage of change, which include precontemplation, contemplation, preparation, action, and maintenance (Joo & Liu, 2021). For Black patients, it is also essential to address the broader social determinants of health—such as neighborhood safety, access to healthy food, and healthcare inequities—that influence readiness and ability to engage in behavior change (Saunders et al., 2016).

THE INTERCONNECTION OF MENTAL HEALTH, STRESS, AND OBESITY IN THE BLACK COMMUNITY

Obesity and mental health are intricately linked, particularly in the Black community, where rates of depression and anxiety are disproportionately high (Brennan & Williams, 2013). Social determinants such as racism, economic instability, and neighborhood violence contribute to chronic stress, which in turn promotes emotional eating and weight gain (Joo & Liu, 2021). To reduce stress levels and optimize mental health, patients may benefit from lifestyle psychiatry, which emphasizes the role of stress management techniques, such as mindfulness, yoga, and exercise, in improving mental health and reducing obesity (Earles et al., 2020).

ADDRESSING CULTURAL STIGMA AND STRUCTURAL BARRIERS TO BEHAVIORAL INTERVENTIONS

Cultural stigma around both mental health and obesity is a significant barrier to participation in weight management programs in the Black community. Many Black individuals perceive weight loss programs as culturally irrelevant or fear being judged by healthcare providers who do not share their cultural background (Hargreaves et al., 2020). Incorporating culturally competent communication, community-based participatory research methods, and engaging trusted community leaders can reduce these barriers and increase program uptake (Lee et al., 2019). Structural barriers, such as lack of insurance and limited access to mental health services, also need to be addressed to ensure equitable treatment access.

TAILORING INTERVENTIONS FOR EATING DISORDERS AND DISORDERED EATING

Disordered eating patterns, such as binge eating, food addiction, and restrictive dieting, are often overlooked in Black patients due to cultural misconceptions and inadequate screening tools (Lee et al., 2019). Addressing these behaviors requires culturally adapted interventions that include nutritional counseling, CBT, and group support (Babatunde et al., 2020). Programs like the Binge Eating Disorder Program at Howard University have successfully incorporated culturally specific strategies to address emotional eating and improve weight management outcomes (Earles et al., 2020).

THE ROLE OF ANTI-OBESITY MEDICATIONS (AOMs) IN TREATING OBESITY AND MENTAL HEALTH IN BLACK PATIENTS

Recent studies have shown that anti-obesity medications, such as GLP-1 receptor agonists, can reduce emotional eating, improve satiety, and promote weight loss, making them effective for patients with both obesity and mental health conditions (Earles et al., 2020). Integrating AOMs into a comprehensive lifestyle medicine plan that includes behavioral interventions and psychiatric care, can lead to better long-term outcomes for Black patients (Saunders et al., 2016).

CONCLUSION

The intersection of mental health and obesity presents unique challenges that require a holistic and culturally informed approach to care, especially within the Black community. Addressing both the psychological and physical components of obesity, including the management of weight-inducing psychiatric medications and the stigma surrounding mental health, is essential for achieving long-term clinical outcomes. By incorporating behavioral therapy, nutritional counseling, and stress management into individualized treatment plans, healthcare providers can effectively disrupt the maladaptive cycle that links obesity with mental health disorders. Community-based programs, trauma-informed care, and lifestyle medicine offer promising approaches for supporting individuals in their pursuit of sustainable wellness. It is crucial to emphasize cultural relevance, respect, and multidisciplinary collaboration to create a healthcare environment that fosters both mental and physical well-being.

CLINICAL CONSIDERATIONS CHECKLIST: CULTIVATING READINESS FOR CHANGE

The readiness for change framework is essential in working with Black patients who may have varying levels of motivation and awareness of obesity-related health risks (Shrivastava & Johnston, 2010). Utilizing the

Transtheoretical Model of Change, which includes stages such as precontemplation, contemplation, preparation, action, and maintenance, allows clinicians to tailor interventions based on the patient's current mindset.

For example, raising awareness and addressing health literacy may be more effective for those in the precontemplation stage, while goal setting and problem-solving strategies would be more suitable for patients in the preparation or action stages (Shrivastava & Johnston, 2010). Culturally sensitive communication, coupled with a deep understanding of the social determinants of health affecting Black communities, can significantly enhance the effectiveness of these interventions.

When considering behavioral interventions for obesity treatment, it is critical to assess the patient's readiness for change before implementing a treatment plan. Incorporating pre-appointment questions can help clinicians gauge a patient's stage of change and identify barriers that may impede progress. The following pre-appointment questions can be used to facilitate a comprehensive assessment.

Pre-Appointment Questions for Readiness and Motivation Assessment

1. *Understanding the Patient's Perspective*
   - How do you feel about your current weight and overall health?
   - Have you attempted weight management programs or lifestyle changes before? If so, what worked and what didn't?
   - What are your primary health and wellness goals (e.g., weight loss, improving mental health, increasing energy)?
2. *Assessing Current Health Behaviors*
   - How would you describe your current eating habits? Do you feel these habits align with your health goals?
   - How often do you engage in physical activity? What types of exercise or activities do you enjoy?
   - Do you feel stress or emotions influence your eating patterns or physical activity?
3. *Exploring Motivation and Barriers*
   - On a scale from 1 to 10, how motivated are you to make changes to your lifestyle to reach your goals?
   - What do you see as the biggest challenge to achieving your health goals?
   - Do you feel that there are any cultural or community-related factors that support or hinder your health efforts?
4. *Support System and Resources*
   - Do you have a support system (family, friends, or a community group) that encourages your health goals?
   - What resources (e.g., dietitian, coach, support groups) have you found helpful or would like to access?

- Are there specific barriers to accessing these resources? (e.g., time, cost, lack of culturally sensitive options)

5. *Psychiatric Considerations*
   - Have you experienced any mental health conditions such as depression, anxiety, or trauma that have affected your weight or eating habits?
   - Are you currently taking any psychiatric medications that might influence your weight? If so, have you noticed any changes in appetite or weight since starting them?
   - Are you open to exploring how mental health and emotional well-being intersect with weight management?

6. *Cultural and Personal Identity*
   - Are there cultural beliefs or practices that influence your eating habits or views on health and body image?
   - How does your cultural or community identity shape your approach to health and wellness?

By using these pre-appointment questions, clinicians can better understand the patient's perspective, tailor interventions to their needs, and foster a more supportive therapeutic alliance that aligns with the patient's values and goals (Kitzman et al., 2021; Brennan & Williams, 2013; Glasgow et al., 2013; Shrivastava & Johnston, 2010).

BEHAVIORAL HEALTH, STIGMA, AND OBESITY QUESTIONNAIRE

1. Do you feel comfortable discussing your weight and mental health concerns with a healthcare provider?
   - Yes
   - No

   If no, what makes it difficult? _____

2. Have you ever felt judged or misunderstood by healthcare professionals when discussing your weight?
   - Yes
   - No

   If yes, please describe: _____

3. Do you believe that mental health and weight issues are linked?
   - Strongly Agree
   - Agree
   - Neutral
   - Disagree
   - Strongly Disagree

4. Have you experienced stigma or negative comments about your weight from family, friends, or in social settings?
   • Yes
   • No
   If yes, how did it impact you? _____

5. How often do you avoid social situations or activities because of your weight or how you feel about your body?
   • Never
   • Rarely
   • Sometimes
   • Often
   • Always

6. Have cultural beliefs or community norms influenced your view of obesity or mental health?
   • Yes
   • No
   If yes, please explain: _____

7. Do you feel pressure to lose weight from family, friends, or community members?
   • Yes
   • No
   If yes, who and how? _____

8. Has a healthcare provider ever addressed weight management in a way that made you feel uncomfortable?
   • Yes
   • No
   If yes, what could have made the conversation better? _____

9. Do you believe weight management should include mental health support?
   • Yes
   • No
   Why or why not? _____

10. Do you find it challenging to talk about the emotional aspects of weight management, such as stress eating, with your doctor?
    • Yes
    • No
    If yes, what would help you feel more comfortable? _____

Chapter 10

Physical Activity for Patients with Obesity

William A.J. Ross, III, William L. Doss, III, MD,
Kathi Earles, MD, MPH, DABOM,
William A.J. Ross, Jr., MD, and
Sylvia Gonsahn-Bollie, MD, DABOM, FOMA

Start where you are. Use what you have. Do what you can.

—Arthur Ashe

Chapter 10 Highlights

- Culturally resonant activities such as line dancing and jumping rope promote both physical health and social engagement. Family and community involvement enhances motivation and sustainability of physical activity programs.
- Black patients with obesity may face specific challenges, such as socioeconomic constraints, lack of safe exercise spaces, and hair care concerns, which must be acknowledged and addressed through personalized, practical exercise recommendations. Each patient's journey is unique and stereotypes should be avoided. Always ask and don't assume.
- Emphasize the long-term health benefits of physical activity, such as improved mental well-being, reduced chronic disease risks, and cardiometabolic benefits, rather than focusing solely on weight loss, fostering greater patient adherence and long-term success.

INTRODUCTION

Physical activity is defined as any movement of the body that contracts skeletal muscle and causes energy expenditure (U.S. Department of Health and Human Services [HHS], 2018). It is well established that purposeful physical activity, or "exercise," is a critical part of obesity management. In addition to contributing to modest weight reduction and weight maintenance, exercise improves emotional well-being, functional ability, and quality sleep. Over time, exercise can improve physical fitness, which is the ability to carry out

DOI: 10.1201/9781032622217-13

tasks with energy and alertness. Improving physical fitness also decreases the risk of death from all causes and the incidence and severity of many chronic diseases. For African Americans, a variety of factors influence the successful implementation of an exercise plan in obesity management to improve physical fitness. In this chapter, purposeful physical activity will be defined and classified, and the risks, benefits, barriers, and facilitators to establishing exercise programs in the U.S. African American community will be discussed. However, several of the principles discussed in this chapter may be applicable to Black people throughout the African Diaspora.

CHARACTERISTICS OF PHYSICAL ACTIVITY

The second edition of the *Physical Activity Guidelines for Americans*, published by the U.S. Department of Health and Human Services (HHS), defines physical fitness as the ability to carry out daily tasks without fatigue and with enough energy to enjoy leisure-time pursuits and respond to emergencies (HHS, 2018). Physical fitness has multiple components, including cardiorespiratory and musculoskeletal fitness, flexibility, balance, and speed, which are summarized in Table 10.1.

All physical activities do not require the same amount of energy. The level of energy required, or intensity, is an important factor in determining how effective an activity will be in improving overall fitness. The amount of energy used by the body for any activity is described as either light, moderate, or vigorous and is defined in metabolic equivalents of task (METs). An MET is the comparison of energy used during any activity to the energy used while at rest. For example, the rate of energy expended while sitting still is 1 MET. Running a mile requires 10 times the amount of energy as sitting still and is therefore rated at 10 METs. An easy way to teach patients to assess if they are performing moderate or vigorous physical activity is the "Sing or

Table 10.1 Components of Physical Fitness

Fitness Component	Description
Cardiorespiratory	Ability to perform large-muscle, whole-body exercise at moderate intensity for an extended period
Musculoskeletal	Combined function of strength, endurance and power to enable performance of work
Flexibility	Range of motion at a joint or group of joints
Balance	Ability to maintain equilibrium while moving or stationary
Speed	Ability to move quickly

Source: Adapted from *Physical Activity Guidelines for Americans* (2nd ed.), by the U.S. Department of Health and Human Services, 2018.

Table 10.2 Physical Activity Intensity Levels

Intensity Level	Definition	Example
Light (Low)	Activities requiring <3 METs	Playing Piano [2 METs]
Moderate	Activities requiring 3–6 METs	Electric Slide; Dancing [4+ METs]
Vigorous	Activities requiring >6 METs	Water Aerobics [7.5 METs]

Source: Adapted from the *Compendium of Physical Activities* (Ainsworth et al., 2011).

Talk" test. Moderate physical activity is defined as moving too rapidly to sing, whereas vigorous physical activity is moving too rapidly to talk during the activity. Table 10.2 summarizes physical activity intensity levels.

BENEFITS OF PHYSICAL ACTIVITY

The amount of weight loss resulting from physical activity, typically averaging 2 kg, is generally modest compared to other obesity interventions (Swift et al., 2014). However, exercise is most beneficial for maintaining weight loss after the initial reduction (Jensen et al., 2024). Growing evidence supports the combination of aerobic and muscle-strengthening exercises to improve body composition during obesity treatment. Specifically, exercise regimens that focus on reducing fat mass while preserving or optimizing lean body mass are referred to as "high-quality" weight loss (Mechanick et al., 2024). For example, aerobic exercises like brisk walking or cycling, combined with muscle-strengthening activities such as resistance training or weight lifting, are effective in achieving this balance.

Health Impacts of Physical Activity

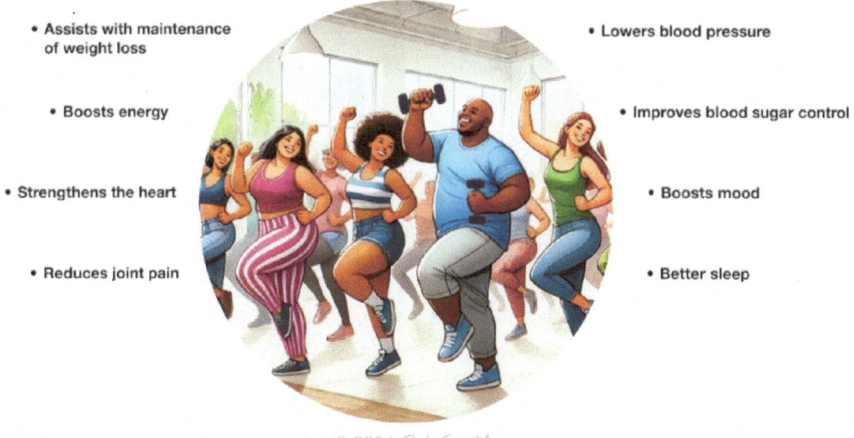

- Assists with maintenance of weight loss
- Boosts energy
- Strengthens the heart
- Reduces joint pain
- Lowers blood pressure
- Improves blood sugar control
- Boosts mood
- Better sleep

© 2024 *Body Scientific*

Table 10.3 Selected Benefits of Physical Activity

Lower risk of death; All causes	Improved quality of life
Lower risk of cardiovascular disease	Improved cognition
Lower risk of hypertension	Improved sleep
Lower risk of type 2 diabetes	Improved bone and joint health
Lower risk of some cancers	Reduced anxiety
Lower risk of falls and fall-related injuries	Reduced symptoms of depression
Lower risk of dementia	Reduced weight

Additionally, substantial evidence shows that regular moderate to vigorous physical activity offers significant health benefits beyond weight loss or high-quality weight reduction. Some of these benefits, such as reduced anxiety, lower blood pressure, improved cognitive function, and better sleep quality, can be experienced almost immediately. Improved sleep, in particular, has a positive effect on weight loss (Papatriantafyllou et al., 2022). Other health benefits, like increased cardiorespiratory fitness, enhanced muscular strength, and reduced symptoms of depression, require consistent, purposeful physical activity over several weeks or months. Furthermore, physical activity can help delay the progression of chronic diseases, many of which are common comorbidities of obesity, such as hypertension and diabetes.

When developing a physical activity–focused obesity treatment plan, it is crucial to highlight these comprehensive benefits to patients. This helps ensure that patients don't become discouraged if the scale does not show rapid changes from exercise alone. Table 10.3 outlines some of the key benefits of physical activity.

EFFECTIVE COMMUNICATION FOR BLACK PATIENTS WITH OBESITY

Communication is a critical factor in successful obesity management. Unfortunately, Black patients with obesity often encounter barriers when interacting with healthcare clinicians. These barriers include communication challenges, patient distrust of the healthcare system, and a lack of shared decision-making, all of which contribute to poor patient engagement.

A study evaluating the quality of clinician communication found that Black patients with obesity were less likely to report that their clinicians facilitated clear, in-depth discussions about obesity and its associated health consequences (Wong et al., 2015). Another study revealed that Black patients with a BMI ≥ 30 kg/m² were less likely to receive an obesity diagnosis compared to White patients with similar BMI levels (Post et al., 2011). Additionally, patients were more likely to receive dietary advice from their clinician if the patient and clinician shared the same race, highlighting the importance of racial concordance in clinician–patient relationships (Bleich et al., 2012).

Empathetic, bias-free communication is essential for effective obesity management and significantly influences patient health outcomes (Phelan et al., 2015). Key elements of empathetic listening—such as maintaining eye contact 50% of the time while speaking and 70% while listening—help foster trust and make patients feel heard. Clinicians should also face their patients, lean forward during the conversation, and sit at the same level to convey attentiveness and respect. These simple yet impactful behaviors can break down communication barriers and build rapport.

Patient-first language and shared decision-making have also been associated with better healthcare outcomes for patients with obesity (Muscat et al., 2021). For example, clinicians can involve patients in setting realistic health goals, which can help them feel empowered in their treatment. It is crucial to discuss the comprehensive benefits of weight management with patients, so they don't become discouraged by slow progress or feel dismissed due to a lack of empathy.

Incorporating these communication strategies into patient interactions can improve engagement and ultimately enhance health outcomes. Table 10.4 lists characteristics and descriptions of empathetic listening skills.

Table 10.4 Empathetic Listening Skills for Assessing and Addressing Barriers to Physical Activity

Empathetic Listening Element	Description
Eye Contact	• Establish eye contact at start of exam • Maintain eye contact 50% of time while speaking • Maintain eye contact 70% of time while listening • Understand cultural influences on eye contact
Body Posture	• Face patient • Lean toward the patient
Body Level	• Sit • Get as close to patient level as is reasonable
Facial Expression	• Smile at start *and* when appropriate • Show concern
Remove Barriers	• Remove hand(s) from door/phone/computer • Avoid initially sitting behind computer • Do not cross arms or legs
Touch	• Extend hand for greeting (when reasonable) • *Always* perform a physical exam • Touch is expected during exam • Absence of touch during evaluation is noticed

CREATING A PLAN

An obesity treatment plan should be personalized and incorporate cultural preferences for activity type. This is particularly true for Black patients with obesity, for whom health outcomes are more significantly influenced by non-medical factors (Ard et al., 2000; Lofton et al., 2023). Current literature indicates that Black patients with obesity who receive a diagnosis and treatment plan from their healthcare clinician are more likely to view their condition as treatable and are more likely to commit to a program to address the disease. Also, Black patients with obesity who had a healthcare provider act as a treatment or accountability partner were much more likely to sustain and complete an obesity management program (Omoisilli et al., 2019). In 2018, the U.S. Preventive Services Task Force noted that the most important factor in successfully addressing obesity was the amount of attention and support individuals received while pursuing their treatment plan, rather than calorie restriction or diet modification (U.S. Preventive Services Task Force, 2018).

The emphasis of a treatment plan for patients with obesity should focus on health gains, not weight loss alone. Befort et al. (2008) found that for a significant number of Black patients with obesity, improved health is a motivating factor for weight loss. Additionally, Ward et al. (2009) found that focusing on the overall health benefits of the treatment plan is an effective motivator for weight loss for Black patients with obesity. Approaches that emphasize weight loss as the only benefit, without addressing associated comorbidities, have a significantly high dropout rate. It is important to remember that weight is just one symptom of obesity, a complex disease associated with more than 200 health conditions.

Overcoming "The Sitting Disease"

A recent study shows that 30% of Black Americans were physically inactive, or sedentary, compared to 23% of non-Hispanic White Americans (Ussery et al., 2018). Sedentary behavior is linked to numerous adverse health effects and diseases that are collectively referred to as "The Sitting Disease." Sedentary behavior is defined by body position—generally reclining or sitting—and a lack of energy expenditure (≤ 1.5 METs). The Sitting Disease causes injury through several mechanisms, including reduced blood flow to the lower extremities and increased inflammatory biomarkers. This combination can lead to obesity, reduced insulin action, metabolic syndrome, and eventually diabetes if left unaddressed. An effective treatment plan for the Sitting Disease includes alternating between sitting and standing every 30 minutes while engaged in sedentary activity.

The *Physical Activity Guidelines for Americans*, published by the U.S. Department of Health and Human Services (HHS, 2018), recommends the following:

- **Aerobic Exercise:** Moderate physical activity for 150 minutes per week or vigorous activity for 75 minutes per week.
- **Muscle Strengthening:** Moderate intensity or greater of all muscle groups at least 2 days per week.

For people with obesity, this combination of aerobic and muscle strengthening exercise is critical to ensure beneficial body composition changes with weight loss (Jensen et al., 2024).

Motivational interviewing techniques, as described in Chapter 6, can be used to initiate the discussion about starting an exercise plan with a patient who has a history of established sedentary habits. Both the clinician and patient may find the significant amount of changes needed to be daunting. The challenge can be reduced by setting small, incremental goals. An achievable first step is to actively decrease sedentary behavior with straightforward and easily doable methods, such as intentionally standing for short periods while working instead of sitting at a desk for extended periods. Early small successes establish the framework for consistent activity with increasing levels of intensity, as appropriate.

Beginning Early

A growing body of literature confirms that the adoption of earlier health-enhancing behaviors provides a greater opportunity to reduce and prevent chronic illnesses that disproportionately affect Black patients with obesity (Krist et al., 2017). In addition to early health-enhancing behaviors like exercise, consistent physical activity has been found to be critical for preventing morbidity and mortality, especially among older adults (Kokkinos, 2012). Population-based studies provide evidence that leisure-time physical activity is a predictor of overall health and physical functioning (Lindström et al., 2023). However, it is never too late to get started. Patients should be encouraged to incorporate tolerable levels of physical activity that correspond with their stage of obesity.

Risks with Exercise

Developing a path to physical fitness requires an awareness of common musculoskeletal injuries and cardiopulmonary issues. Injury during exercise is related to the gap between a patient's usual level of activity and a higher level of intensity (Campbell et al., 2012). Understanding these risks allows for a personalized approach in an exercise prescription aimed at minimizing injuries and maximizing adherence to a healthier lifestyle.

Self-Administered Risk Assessment

The Physical Activity Readiness Questionnaire (PAR-Q) is a resource to determine the level of risk for those desiring a purposeful activity program. The questionnaire is based on several exercise-induced health considerations. Positive answers documented on any of the questions below require an evaluation by a healthcare clinician before initiating a purposeful physical activity program.

Sample PAR-Q Questions

1. Has your doctor ever said that you have a heart condition and that you should only perform physical activity recommended by a doctor?
2. Do you feel pain in your chest during physical activity?
3. In the past month, have you had chest pain when not performing physical activity?
4. Do you lose balance because of dizziness, or do you ever lose consciousness?
5. Do you have a bone or joint problem that could be made worse by a change in your physical activity?
6. Is your doctor currently prescribing drugs (e.g., water pills) for your blood pressure or heart condition?
7. Do you know of any other reason why you should not engage in physical activity?

(Adapted from Shepard, R. J. (2014). A brief history of exercise and physical activity participation clearance and prescription: 2. Canadian contributions to the development of objective, evidence-based procedures. *Health and Fitness Journal of Canada*, 7(1), 36–68.)

BARRIERS TO PHYSICAL ACTIVITY

Addressing Barriers to Exercise

Black patients with obesity are less likely to engage in physical activity compared to other racial groups (Lofton et al., 2023). Barriers to physical activity among Black women with obesity include a lack of awareness of effective exercise techniques, safe and suitable locations, cost of exercise programs, inaccessible facilities, transportation challenges, and health concerns (Joseph et al., 2015). However, increased motivation and exercise participation have been associated with factors such as family interaction and community connection (Gothe & Kendall, 2016). Clinicians should be mindful that each individual's experience is unique and stereotypes should be avoided. It is essential to ask about the patient's specific barriers rather than making assumptions.

Physical Activity and Social Determinants of Health (SDOH)

As discussed in Chapter 4, "The Role of Social Determinants of Health on the Disease of Obesity," SDOH influences all aspects of health, including physical activity. Black people, who are disproportionately affected by lower socioeconomic status, often face significant socioeconomic barriers when it comes to exercise. For instance, recommending a gym membership may be counterproductive for a patient with obesity who faces economic constraints. Other demands, such as working multiple jobs, caregiving, or educational responsibilities, may leave little time or energy for exercise. In these cases, incorporating family members into physical activity, either as participants or accountability partners, can help shift the focus from binary decision-making (e.g., family vs. exercise) to considering multiple options.

Additionally, access to safe outdoor spaces for walking may be limited in certain communities. In these cases, modifying the exercise plan to include safe, accessible options, like climbing stairs in an apartment building or following an app-guided home exercise routine, should be considered.

Prior Injuries and Physical Conditions

Reduced physical fitness and prior injuries are additional barriers to exercise. Past injuries, especially to the same body part, can increase the risk of re-injury. This risk can be minimized by setting appropriate personal goals and engaging in a variety of physical activities to prevent overuse injuries. Before starting an exercise regimen, it is crucial to address previous injuries and implement strategies for preventing further injury.

Furthermore, obesity-related conditions such as osteoarthritis and obesity hypoventilation syndrome can make physical activity more challenging. For patients with severe obesity, focusing on reducing body weight by at least 5% before intensifying an exercise regimen may be necessary. However, low-intensity exercise is not synonymous with inactivity. For example, chair exercises or low-impact aerobic activities can serve as effective alternatives to high-intensity workouts.

Competing Demands and Time Constraints

Many African American women are aware of the importance of physical activity and can articulate its benefits, even if they are not currently engaged in regular exercise (James et al., 2015). Common barriers include busy lifestyles, lack of time, and arriving home too late to exercise. Women, particularly mothers who work outside of the home, often feel conflicted between dedicating time to physical activity and spending time with their families (Fallon et al., 2005). These barriers affect women of all body sizes, not just those with obesity.

Health educators can address these concerns by emphasizing short workouts that can be done at home and recommending fitness apps. Additionally, encouraging family-based activities offers a practical, inclusive way to engage in physical activity without sacrificing family time.

Hair Considerations

A study by Hall et al. (2013) revealed that Black women frequently avoid physical activity due to concerns about the impact of sweat on their hairstyles. Maintaining hairstyles can be time-consuming and expensive, and regular exercise can lead to hair damage or loss (Versey, 2014). Nearly 38% of Black women in the study reported avoiding physical activity due to hair-related concerns, and those who identified hair as a barrier were almost three times less likely to meet national physical activity guidelines (Rettner, 2012).

These concerns are not merely vanity but are often rooted in systemic racism. Black women's hair has historically been a source of discrimination, especially in the workplace. Legislative efforts, such as the CROWN Act (2024), aim to prevent discrimination based on natural hair, but only 27 of 50 states have passed the law at the time of writing (CROWN Act, 2024). Thus, the need for "socially acceptable" hairstyles remains a realistic consideration for many Black women, which can impede their ability to exercise. Fortunately, products like GymWrap by Nicole Ari Parker™ have been developed to help preserve hairstyles during exercise.

Culturally Resonant Physical Activity

To ensure lasting engagement in physical activity, it is essential to incorporate culturally resonant activities. Collaborative exercises like line dancing (e.g., "Electric Slide") or jumping rope not only provide moderate to vigorous physical activity but also foster community engagement and social support. Participating in or creating community-led initiatives, with support from family, friends, and neighbors, significantly boosts motivation and accountability, leading to improved health outcomes for Black patients with obesity.

Success stories from peers or role models from similar backgrounds can also serve as powerful motivators.

Historically, the Black community has often gathered to improve health. For example, Professor Ava Purkiss's book *Fit Citizens* highlights how Black women have collectively promoted exercise throughout history. Modern groups such as GirlTrek™ and Black Girls Run™ have gathered thousands of Black women to improve health and foster community through walking and running. Similarly, Black Men Run™ and the African American Male Wellness Agency™ offer opportunities for Black men to engage in fitness while promoting overall well-being.

Body Image and Cultural Norms

Cultural perceptions about body image and size may also influence physical activity planning. In some Black communities, a fuller body is viewed positively, which can reduce the perceived need for weight loss. This cultural acceptance of body size can affect the motivation to start and maintain a physical activity program. Shifting the focus from weight loss to fitness and disease prevention is crucial to overcoming this potential barrier. Chapter 5, "Weight Bias and Cultural Attitudes toward Obesity," delves further into how cultural perceptions impact obesity management.

MONITORING AND ADJUSTMENTS

Regular follow-ups with healthcare clinicians are crucial to ensuring safe and effective physical activity regimens, leading to better adherence. Frequent communication regarding the type, consistency, and patient experience positively impacts healthcare outcomes. With the use of telemedicine platforms and wearable technology, physical activity programs can be monitored remotely in real-time, helping to ensure proper execution and continued participation (Haleem et al., 2021). It is important to note that technology should supplement, not replace, consultations with clinicians.

By incorporating strategies such as regular monitoring, injury prevention, and the creation of supportive, culturally sensitive environments, individuals can enhance their exercise experience and cultivate long-term sustainability.

CONCLUSION

Incorporating physical activity into the management of obesity is essential not only for weight loss but also for achieving long-term health benefits, including improved cardiovascular health, mental well-being, and functional mobility.

Physical activity, when approached with gradual progression and cultural sensitivity, can empower patients to make sustainable changes. For Black patients with obesity, understanding the unique barriers such as socioeconomic challenges, cultural body image norms, and hair care concerns are critical in crafting personalized, supportive, and sustainable exercise programs. Clinicians should encourage patients by emphasizing that physical activity is a lifelong commitment, focusing on overall health gains rather than weight loss alone. By fostering empathetic, bias-free communication and leveraging culturally resonant physical activity, healthcare providers can motivate patients to embrace fitness as part of their daily lives, overcoming the challenges of "The Sitting Disease" and improving both physical and mental health outcomes.

CLINICAL CONSIDERATIONS CHECKLIST: PHYSICAL ACTIVITY FOR BLACK PATIENTS WITH OBESITY

Key Discussion Points	Suggested Approach
Start the Conversation	*"Start where you are. Use what you have. Do what you can."*—Arthur Ashe • Ask patients about their current level of physical activity and any barriers they face. • Avoid assumptions and let them share their unique experiences.
Explore Culturally Resonant Activities	• Discuss culturally relevant options such as line dancing (e.g., "Electric Slide") or jumping rope, which promote both physical health and community engagement.
Address Barriers	• Common barriers among Black patients with obesity include: Safe, accessible exercise spaces, cost of programs or transportation, and hair care concerns. • Ask the patient to identify which barriers they personally face, and provide practical alternatives (e.g., indoor walking, app-guided workouts, products like GymWrap).
Highlight the Benefits beyond Weight Loss	• Emphasize long-term benefits of physical activity, such as improved mental well-being, better sleep quality, reduced risk of chronic diseases like hypertension and diabetes, and enhanced functional mobility. • Avoid focusing solely on weight loss to foster greater adherence.
Incorporate Family and Community	• Encourage patients to involve family members and the community in their exercise plan. This can increase motivation and sustainability. • Family members can participate in activities or serve as accountability partners.

(Continued)

(Continued)

Key Discussion Points	Suggested Approach
Personalized Exercise Recommendations	• Consider the patient's unique situation: socioeconomic factors (e.g., gym access), health conditions (e.g., osteoarthritis), and cultural norms around body image. • Suggest activities that can be done at home or in the community, such as stair climbing or low-impact chair exercises.
Monitor and Adjust	• Use telemedicine platforms and wearable technology to monitor progress and adjust plans as needed. • Regular follow-ups improve adherence and help prevent injury. • Ensure that technology supplements do not replace consultations with clinicians. • Utilize in-person visits as needed.
Set Realistic, Achievable Goals	• Break down goals into small, manageable steps to build consistency. • Encourage patients to celebrate progress, even small wins. • Example: "Let's start with standing more during the day and work toward more regular movement."
Encourage Open Communication	• Ask patients how they feel about their exercise experience and any adjustments they need. • This builds trust and keeps them engaged in the process. • Remind patients that physical activity should feel sustainable and enjoyable.

Chapter 11

Pharmacotherapy for Obesity Treatment

William L. Doss,
Tiffani Bell-Washington, MD, MPH, MBA, FAPA,
FOMA, DABOM, DABLM, and
Kathi Earles, MD, MPH, DABOM

> I had an awareness of [weight loss] medications, but felt I had to prove I had the willpower to do it. I now no longer feel that way.
>
> —Oprah Winfrey, in *People* Magazine, December 2023

Chapter 11 Highlights

- **Historical and Systemic Barriers:** Black communities have long faced major obstacles to receiving fair healthcare. Racial biases affect how easily they can access treatment. These issues come from the idea of race as a social construct and are supported by a history of injustice, such as surgical experiments done on enslaved people. Today, disparities still exist, like the insufficient treatment of pain for Black patients.
- **Impact of Anti-Obesity Medications:** Even with these challenges, anti-obesity medications have been recognized as useful tools for managing obesity and reducing related health problems. These medications work in different ways, such as increasing hormones that make a person feel full or reducing fat absorption in the body, which helps with weight loss and overall health improvement.
- **Diversity of Treatment Options:** This chapter explores various medications aimed at treating obesity, including those designed for specific genetic conditions. Although some medications may not work well for everyone, others show good results in controlling appetite and managing weight. This suggests that personalized treatment plans are important for effectively addressing obesity in Black communities.

INTRODUCTION

Throughout history, Black communities have faced significant barriers in accessing equitable healthcare, many of which are rooted in the understanding of race as a social construct. This construct was historically used to justify

DOI: 10.1201/9781032622217-14

slavery, despite the lack of genetic differences between racial groups. As discussed in Chapter 1, "Who Is Black?" the completion of the 2003 Human Genome Project confirmed that race lacks a genetic basis, revealing that humans are 99% identical at the DNA level (Duello et al., 2021). However, despite these scientific findings, racial bias remains pervasive in healthcare, contributing to disparities in access to essential treatments, including anti-obesity medications.

This chapter will explore the historical context of medication use in Black communities, highlight key FDA-approved anti-obesity medications, and examine how social determinants of health (SDOH) influence access to care. In doing so, the chapter emphasizes the importance of addressing systemic inequities to ensure equitable treatment and improved health outcomes for those disproportionately affected by obesity.

HISTORICAL CONSIDERATIONS FOR MEDICATION USE IN THE BLACK COMMUNITY

Supportive evidence can be traced as far back as surgical experiments performed by a White 19th-century surgeon on enslaved Black women without anesthesia to explore techniques for traumatic post-delivery vaginal fistulas (Wall, 2006). Twentieth-century examples include the COVID-related death of Dr. Susan Moore following the dismissal of her requests for pain medication due to the perception that her Black skin provided a higher tolerance for pain and assumed drug-seeking behavior. Examples also exist when diagnosing and treating Black patients with obesity, including the failure to provide education on lifestyle modification, medication use, or surgery referral when appropriate (Byrd et al., 2018). Despite these issues, interventions for managing obesity, including the use of anti-obesity medications, have been shown to not only reduce weight but also lower many associated comorbidities (Lofton et al., 2023).

CURRENT FDA-APPROVED OBESITY PHARMACOLOGICAL TREATMENTS

Many pharmaceutical agents treat obesity by inducing weight reduction ("weight loss") through stimulating the secretion of satiety hormones or inhibiting the absorption of dietary fat (Brandfon et al., 2023). Additional obesity pharmacotherapy is available to treat genetic-related causes of obesity, such as Bardet-Biedl syndrome and proopiomelanocortin (POMC) deficiency, albeit with limited efficacy. Products targeting melanocortin-4 receptors (MC4R) and leptin have been developed to restore the function of these receptors, resulting in normal regulation of appetite and energy balance.

Table 11.1 provides an overview of the FDA-approved obesity pharmacological* treatments. The current FDA term for obesity pharmacological treatments is "anti-obesity medications" (AOMs), similar to anti-hypertensives or anti-hyperglycemics. However, given the prevalence of weight bias, the term "anti-obesity medication" may have a connotation that is not perceived with other types of medications. As the field of obesity medicine evolves, the term "anti-obesity medication" should be revised. Yet, for the sake of common language, anti-obesity medication or AOM will be used in this chapter, with the need to be medically accurate but not as a form of weight bias.

BENEFITS OF ANTI-OBESITY TREATMENT

As an adjunct to lifestyle management and behavior modification, AOMs offer an option to achieve significant weight loss (>5%) and improve health outcomes. Several FDA-approved AOMs have demonstrated impactful weight loss and the ability to reduce the risk of several associated comorbidities, including type 2 diabetes, cardiovascular disease, and cerebrovascular accidents. Sustained weight loss has also been associated with improved insulin sensitivity, reduced inflammation, and a reduction in blood pressure, which are all contributing factors to many obesity-associated comorbidities. Additionally, obesity is associated with at least 13 types of cancers, including adenocarcinoma, postmenopausal breast, colorectal, endometrial, and gallbladder cancers (Pati et al., 2023).

RACIAL BARRIERS AND ETHNIC DISPARITIES IN ANTI-OBESITY MEDICATION ACCESS

Despite the positive benefits of many newly developed AOMs, access remains low for AOMs in the general population. Access to AOMs is even lower in Black and Brown communities, despite having the highest prevalence of obesity and many of its comorbidities. Contributing factors obstructing access to AOMs include a lack of insurance, inconsistent access to care, low family income, lower levels of education, and the bias and stigma associated with the disease of obesity (Ruan et al., 2024).

Although the Affordable Care Act was passed in 2010, ten states did not expand Medicaid, including Alabama, Florida, Georgia, Kansas, Mississippi, South Carolina, Tennessee, Texas, Wisconsin, and Wyoming. Many of these states have some of the highest rates of obesity. Additionally, a significant percentage of Medicaid beneficiaries are Black and Brown, who also have the highest obesity rates in the nation. Table 11.2 lists the 2024 Medicaid coverage for obesity treatment, including AOMs in selected states as well as the rate of type 2 diabetes and obesity.

Table 11.1 FDA-Approved Anti-Obesity Medications

Drugs	Mechanism of Action	Side Effects	Drug Interactions	Contraindications	% Approximate Placebo Subtracted Weight Loss
Phentermine	Sympathomimetic/ Suppresses appetite	Headache, high blood pressure, palpitations, dry mouth, Insomnia	Potential interactions w/sympathomimetics, alcohol, adrenergic neuron-blocking drugs	Approved for short-term use ONLY CVD Uncontrolled HTN, glaucoma, Hx drug abuse, agitated states, pregnancy	4.4% at 28 weeks
Orlistat	Intestinal lipase inhibitor Reduces fat absorption	Oily stool Flatulence Malabsorption of vitamins A, D, E, K	Oral contraceptives, Cyclosporine, Seizure meds, Thyroid hormones, Warfarin	Chronic malabsorption syndrome Pregnancy	3.8%
Phentermine/ Topiramate	Combination sympathomimetic and carbonic anhydrase inhibitor	Paresthesia, dysgeusia, cleft lip/palate in pregnancy, Insomnia, Dry mouth, Suicidal behavior, Cognitive impairment, Increased HR, Metabolic acidosis, elevated creatinine, decreased blood glucose when on anti-diabetic med, topiramate is teratogen	n/a	Glaucoma Pregnancy (cleft palate)	8.6%

(Continued)

Table 11.1 FDA-Approved Anti-Obesity Medications (Continued)

Drugs	Mechanism of Action	Side Effects	Drug Interactions	Contraindications	% Approximate Placebo Subtracted Weight Loss
Bupropion/ Naltrexone	Combination dopamine/ NE re-uptake inhibitor Mu-opioid receptor antagonist	Nausea, constipation, headache, vomiting, dizziness, acute angle glaucoma, increased risk of suicidal ideation Not for use with uncontrolled HTN, seizures, or alcohol withdrawal	May have drug interactions with opioids, anti-seizure meds, MAO inhibitors, CNS toxicity can occur when using dopaminergic meds	Uncontrolled hypertension Seizure disorder Pregnancy	4.8%
Liraglutide 3.0	GLP-1 agonist (slows gastric emptying, decreases appetite, increases satiety)	N/V, dyspepsia, constipation, diarrhea, fatigue, dizziness, abdominal pain, increased lipase, renal insufficiency May slow absorption in concomitantly administered oral meds, hypoglycemia with sulfonylurea or insulin, pancreatitis	Slows gastric emptying and may impact absorption of concomitantly administered medications, may reduce efficacy of birth control pills	Patient or family with Hx MTC Type 2 MEN pregnancy Precautions in acute pancreatitis, gallbladder disease, diabetic retinopathy, suicidal behavior, associated with hypoglycemia in patients with Type 2 on hypoglycemic agents	5.4%
Semaglutide 2.4 mg	Weekly GLP-1 agonist (slows gastric emptying)	As above	As above	As above	15% at 15 months

(Continued)

Table 11.1 (Continued)

Drugs	Mechanism of Action	Side Effects	Drug Interactions	Contraindications	% Approximate Placebo Subtracted Weight Loss
Tirzepatide	Dual GLP-1-GIP agonist, increases satiety, decreases appetite	As above	As above	Medullary thyroid cancer, MEN, pregnancy	17.8%
Setmelanotide	MC4R agonist	Hyperpigmentation, Nausea, Fatigue	n/a	Diarrhea, Nausea, Headache, Hyperpigmentation	Use in patients >6 years with monogenic or syndromic obesity due to POMC, PCSK1, or LEPR deficiency confirmed by genetic testing
Gelesis 100 (considered a medical device)	Superabsorbent hydrogel particles of cellulose-citric acid matrix Increased fullness	Diarrhea, Abdominal distension and pain, Constipation, Flatulence	n/a	Pregnancy, Chronic malabsorption syndrome, Cholestasis	2% at 6 months

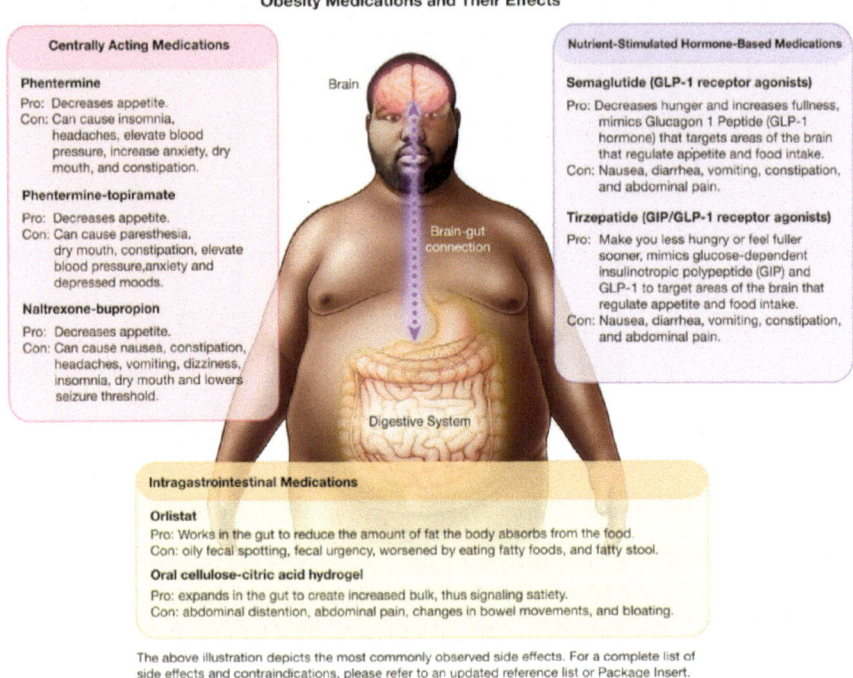

Obesity Medications and Their Effects

Centrally Acting Medications

Phentermine
Pro: Decreases appetite.
Con: Can cause insomnia, headaches, elevate blood pressure, increase anxiety, dry mouth, and constipation.

Phentermine-topiramate
Pro: Decreases appetite.
Con: Can cause paresthesia, dry mouth, constipation, elevate blood pressure, anxiety and depressed moods.

Naltrexone-bupropion
Pro: Decreases appetite.
Con: Can cause nausea, constipation, headaches, vomiting, dizziness, insomnia, dry mouth and lowers seizure threshold.

Brain

Brain-gut connection

Digestive System

Nutrient-Stimulated Hormone-Based Medications

Semaglutide (GLP-1 receptor agonists)
Pro: Decreases hunger and increases fullness, mimics Glucagon 1 Peptide (GLP-1 hormone) that targets areas of the brain that regulate appetite and food intake.
Con: Nausea, diarrhea, vomiting, constipation, and abdominal pain.

Tirzepatide (GIP/GLP-1 receptor agonists)
Pro: Make you less hungry or feel fuller sooner, mimics glucose-dependent insulinotropic polypeptide (GIP) and GLP-1 to target areas of the brain that regulate appetite and food intake.
Con: Nausea, diarrhea, vomiting, constipation, and abdominal pain.

Intragastrointestinal Medications

Orlistat
Pro: Works in the gut to reduce the amount of fat the body absorbs from the food.
Con: oily fecal spotting, fecal urgency, worsened by eating fatty foods, and fatty stool.

Oral cellulose-citric acid hydrogel
Pro: expands in the gut to create increased bulk, thus signaling satiety.
Con: abdominal distention, abdominal pain, changes in bowel movements, and bloating.

The above illustration depicts the most commonly observed side effects. For a complete list of side effects and contraindications, please refer to an updated reference list or Package Insert.

© 2024 Body Scientific

OUT-OF-POCKET COSTS

In addition to the lack of widespread coverage for AOMs, out-of-pocket costs in the United States are prohibitive for many patients who bear a disproportionate burden of obesity. For example, the out-of-pocket cash price for Semaglutide, one of the most effective AOMs, can exceed $1,000 per month in the United States, compared to lower prices in other countries (Ruan et al., 2024). The role of Pharmacy Benefit Managers (PBMs), a unique feature of the U.S. healthcare system, adds to the cost disparity (Mattingly et al., 2023).

In addition to the lack of widespread coverage for AOMs, the out-of-pocket cash price in the United States is cost prohibitive for many patients who bear a disproportionate burden of the disease of obesity (Table 11.3).

In a study by Ruan et al. (2024), evidence confirmed that Black and Brown adult patients had the highest eligibility for Semaglutide at slightly greater than 56.5%. Additionally, Black and Brown patients had a lower family income, were less likely to be insured, or receive consistent healthcare. Notable advancements in obesity treatment have the potential to provide equitable solutions to the obesity epidemic, but inequitable access would only serve to exacerbate existing disparities (Wright et al., 2023).

Table 11.2 2024 Medicaid Obesity Coverage Extracted from the STOP Obesity Alliance

States	Anti-Obesity Medications (AOMs)	Intensive Behavioral Therapy	Metabolic and Bariatric Surgery	Nutritional Counseling	Obesity Prevalence	Type 2 Diabetes Rate
Alabama	Not covered	Covered with limitations	Covered with limitations	Not covered	38.3%	15.5%
Florida	Not covered	Covered with limitations	N/A	Not covered	31.6%	12.2%
Georgia	Not covered	Covered with limitations	N/A	Not covered	37%	12.1%
Kansas	Covered with restrictions and limitations	Covered with restrictions and limitations	Covered with limitations	Not covered	35.7%	11.4%
Mississippi	Covered with restrictions and limitations	Covered with limitations	Not covered	Not covered	39.5%	15.3
South Carolina	Not covered	Covered	Covered with restrictions	Covered	35%	12.9%
Texas	Not covered	Covered with limitations	Covered with limitations and restrictions	Not covered	35.5%	13.9%
Tennessee	Not covered	Covered with limitations	Covered with limitations and restrictions	Not covered	34.1%	12.1%
Wyoming	Not covered	Covered with limitations	Covered with limitations and restrictions	Covered	34.4%	9.3%
Wisconsin	Covered with limitations and restrictions	Covered with limitations	Covered with limitations and restrictions	Not covered	37.7%	10.3%

* Coverage reflects availability at time of publication.

Table 11.3 Out-of-Pocket Cash Price for FDA-Approved Anti-Obesity Medications

Drug	Highest U.S. Price	Lowest National Price	Estimated % Weight Loss
Orlistat	$100	$1 (Vietnam)	8.8%
Naltrexone/Bupropion	$326	$56 (South Africa)	6.4%
Topiramate/Phentermine	$199	$1.3 (Kenya)	9.8%
Semaglutide (oral)	$578	$65 (India)	5.8%
Semaglutide (SQ)	$1350	$95 (Turkey)	14.9%
Liraglutide (SQ)	$1418	$252 (Norway)	8%
Tirzepatide (SQ)	$1070	$715 (U.S. Vets)	20.9%

A study analyzing the eligibility for Semaglutide between 2015 and 2020 found that Black adults had the highest eligibility for the AOM according to Food and Drug Administration criteria. However, they were significantly more likely to lack a consistent source of care, higher education, or health insurance (Ruan et al., 2024). Of note, health insurance coverage in general was not universally indicative of anti-obesity medication coverage due to limitations imposed by a significant proportion of health insurance companies.

In addition to the lack of health insurance coverage, the out-of-pocket cost for AOMs with the greatest efficacy is prohibitive for many patients who need them the most. The higher list price for AOMs in the United States compared to other countries supports the role of the Pharmacy Benefit Manager (PBM), a unique feature in the United States. PBMs serve as intermediaries between pharmacies, plan sponsors (such as insurance companies), employers, pharmaceutical manufacturers, and drug wholesalers (Mattingly et al., 2023). PBMs create formularies, process claims, establish pharmacy networks, review drug utilization, and manage mail-order medications with manufacturers. Additionally, PBMs retain a significant portion of the cash list price and are paid by the insurance company for managing drug costs and by the manufacturer for preferred placement of the product, known as rebates (Mattingly et al., 2023).

Moreover, PBMs are financially compensated by the health plan and receive administrative fees from pharmacies, which are imposed after a patient purchase. Currently, three PBMs control 80% of the prescription drug market, and the largest PBMs and insurers are owned by the same healthcare company. The role of PBMs, unique to the United States, has been implicated in the higher cost of prescription medications when compared to other countries (Mattingly et al., 2023).

CONCLUSION

In summary, the development and availability of anti-obesity medications marks significant progress in the treatment of obesity, offering individuals new opportunities for weight management and the reduction of related health risks. However, persistent disparities in access to these medications, particularly for Black and Brown communities, highlight the need for systemic change. The high cost of medications, limited insurance coverage, and structural biases within the healthcare system remain substantial barriers. Addressing these inequities will require coordinated efforts from healthcare providers, pharmaceutical companies, policymakers, and researchers to ensure that advancements in obesity care do not further widen existing disparities. By prioritizing equitable access and personalized care, the potential of anti-obesity medications can be fully realized, ultimately improving health outcomes and quality of life for all individuals impacted by obesity.

CLINICAL CONSIDERATIONS CHECKLIST: SELECTING ANTI-OBESITY MEDICATIONS FOR THE BLACK COMMUNITY

This guide is designed to support clinicians and patients, especially in the Black community, in selecting personalized anti-obesity medications by addressing unique health needs, cultural considerations, and systemic barriers. It encourages open dialogue about preferences, access challenges, and lifestyle compatibility to develop a collaborative treatment plan that promotes sustainable weight management and equitable care.

Step	Action	Details/Key Questions
1. Assess Health and Lifestyle	Review medical history, comorbidities (e.g., hypertension, diabetes), and cultural barriers to care.	"Have you tried weight loss programs or medications before? What worked or didn't?" "Do you have any concerns about medication side effects or safety?"
2. Explain Medication Options	Provide an overview of FDA-approved medications, with emphasis on relevance to common conditions in Black patients (e.g., hypertension, type 2 diabetes).	Examples: • Orlistat (fat absorption) • Semaglutide/Liraglutide (satiety) • Phentermine/Topiramate (appetite suppression) • "How do you feel about medications that may affect appetite or digestion?"

(Continued)

(Continued)

Step	Action	Details/Key Questions
3. Explore Preferences and Daily Routine	Identify preferred medication type (oral vs. injectable) and assess daily routines to improve adherence.	"Would you prefer a once-daily pill or a weekly injection?" "How can we make medication use easy to fit into your lifestyle?"
4. Address SDOH and Access	Discuss barriers such as insurance, high medication costs, pharmacy access, and systemic bias.	"Do you face any challenges with insurance or access to the pharmacy?" "What support can help you overcome barriers, such as transportation or cost?"
5. Develop a Personalized Plan	Collaborate to select a medication aligned with the patient's health goals and set realistic expectations.	"What are your primary health and weight loss goals?" "Would you feel comfortable scheduling a follow-up soon to assess your progress?"

Chapter 12

Bariatric Surgery
Challenges and Benefits for the Black Community

Shani Belgrave-Heath, MD, FASMBS,
Bria Neomie Woodard, and
Sylvia Gonsahn-Bollie, MD, DABOM, FOMA

Bariatric surgery is highly effective and safe, with patients typically losing 60% of excess body weight after sleeve gastrectomy and 70% after gastric bypass. The risk of serious complications, such as leaks (1%) and death (0.09–0.2%), is very low.

—Amirian et al., 2020

Chapter 12 Highlights

- **Metabolic and bariatric surgery is highly effective and safe:** Patients typically lose 60% of excess body weight after sleeve gastrectomy and 70% after Roux-en-Y gastric bypass. The risk of serious complications from bariatric surgery with sleeve gastrectomy or gastric bypass, such as leaks (1%) and death (0.09–0.2%), is very low.
- **Different bariatric procedures offer distinct benefits and risks:** While sleeve gastrectomy and Roux-en-Y gastric bypass are the most common, less frequently performed surgeries like the duodenal switch provide superior weight loss but come with a higher rate of complications.
- **Racial disparities in metabolic and bariatric surgery outcomes remain a critical concern:** Black patients experience higher rates of early post-surgical complications and less weight loss compared to White patients. Healthcare systems urgently need to adopt more equitable and culturally sensitive care approaches to improve outcomes.

INTRODUCTION

This chapter provides a comprehensive overview of metabolic and bariatric surgery (MBS), detailing its effectiveness, safety, and the variety of procedures available. It explains that bariatric surgery, including sleeve gastrectomy and

DOI: 10.1201/9781032622217-15

Roux-en-Y gastric bypass, can lead to significant weight loss and improve obesity-related conditions such as diabetes, hypertension, and sleep apnea. The chapter also highlights potential complications, such as gastroesophageal reflux disease (GERD) and nutrient deficiencies, while noting the generally low risk of serious outcomes. Additionally, it discusses the cosmetic considerations of massive weight loss, such as excess skin, and the role of body contouring surgeries.

A key focus is on racial and ethnic disparities in MBS outcomes, addressing the higher complication rates and reduced weight loss experienced by Black patients. The chapter emphasizes the importance of addressing these disparities through more equitable healthcare practices and culturally sensitive care, making it a well-rounded resource for understanding both the clinical and social aspects of MBS.

GENERAL CONSIDERATIONS FOR BARIATRIC SURGERY

MBS is safe and durable. Patients can expect to lose approximately 60% of excess body weight after sleeve gastrectomy and 70% after gastric bypass. The leak rate is low, estimated at about 1% for primary bariatric procedures, and the risk of death is very low, estimated at 0.09% to 0.2% (Amirian et al., 2020). MBS is as safe as laparoscopic cholecystectomy (gallbladder removal), a common procedure. Patients often experience improvement or resolution of comorbid conditions, including diabetes, hypertension, dyslipidemia, and sleep apnea. The transformation associated with weight loss surgery also leads to an improved quality of life (American Society for Metabolic and Bariatric Surgery, 2022a).

Qualifications for Weight Loss Surgery

As described in previous chapters, BMI is calculated by dividing a person's weight in kilograms by the square of their height in meters (kg/m^2). From 1991 to 2022, eligibility for MBS was based on a BMI ≥40 kg/m^2 or a BMI ≥35 kg/m^2 with weight-related conditions such as diabetes, hypertension, or sleep apnea. In 2022, guidelines were updated to recommend that MBS be considered for individuals with:

- Metabolic disease and a BMI of 30–34.9 kg/m^2*
- A BMI of 35 kg/m^2 or higher, regardless of the presence, absence, or severity of obesity-related conditions
- BMI thresholds should be adjusted for the Asian population, where a BMI of 25 kg/m^2 suggests clinical obesity, and individuals with a BMI of 27.5 kg/m^2 should be offered MBS (American Society for Metabolic and Bariatric Surgery, 2022)

In the United States, insurance coverage varies, and as of this writing, most coverage is still based on the 1991 criteria for MBS, which are more restrictive than the 2022 guidelines. As of 2022, only about 1% of all qualified patients undergo MBS (Clapp et al., 2024). MBS may feel even more intimidating for non-Hispanic Black patients, who face higher rates of post-surgical complications, hospital readmissions, and less weight loss after surgery (Welsh et al., 2020). Additionally, if a non-Hispanic Black patient has personally witnessed someone struggle with MBS complications or experienced lower efficacy after MBS, it may influence their decision to pursue MBS, especially considering the significant influence of family and peer health recommendations in the Black community.

PRE-OPERATIVE MANAGEMENT BEFORE METABOLIC AND BARIATRIC SURGERY (MBS)

According to the American Society for Metabolic and Bariatric Surgery (ASMBS) 2022 guidelines, pre-operative management is crucial for optimizing patient outcomes in MBS. Before surgery, patients undergo thorough medical, nutritional, and psychological evaluations to assess their readiness and minimize risks. This includes assessments of cardiopulmonary health, comorbid conditions such as diabetes, hypertension, and sleep apnea, as well as identifying nutritional deficiencies in key vitamins and minerals like iron, vitamins D and B12, which can be affected after recovery. Psychological evaluations help determine if patients are mentally prepared for the significant lifestyle changes required post-surgery. Counseling may be recommended to address issues such as emotional eating or eating disorders. Smoking cessation and monitoring of alcohol use are also emphasized, as these can impact healing and post-surgical outcomes.

In addition to these evaluations, patients are often encouraged to lose weight before surgery, as even modest weight loss can reduce liver size and lower surgical risks. Comprehensive lab work, including a complete blood count, comprehensive metabolic panel, thyroid panel, HbA1c, and lipid panel, is necessary to assess overall health and metabolic conditions. Pulmonary function tests and exercise stress tests are performed to ensure the heart and lungs are prepared for surgery.

Some insurance plans require additional pre-operative steps, such as documented weight loss visits, clearance from a primary care provider, and approval from a licensed psychologist. These requirements, while intended to ensure patient safety, can disproportionately disadvantage Black patients and other marginalized groups due to existing healthcare disparities, including limited access to medical resources, insurance coverage, and culturally competent care. Addressing these barriers is essential for creating a more equitable healthcare system that allows all patients to benefit from MBS.

CURRENT TYPES OF METABOLIC AND BARIATRIC SURGERY AND PROCEDURES

Overview

The sleeve gastrectomy and gastric bypass are the most commonly performed MBS procedures. In 2022, the number of MBS procedures was estimated at 280,000, with 90% of those being either sleeve gastrectomies or laparoscopic Roux-en-Y gastric bypasses. Sleeve gastrectomy was performed three times more commonly than Roux-en-Y gastric bypass (American Society for Metabolic and Bariatric Surgery, 2022b).

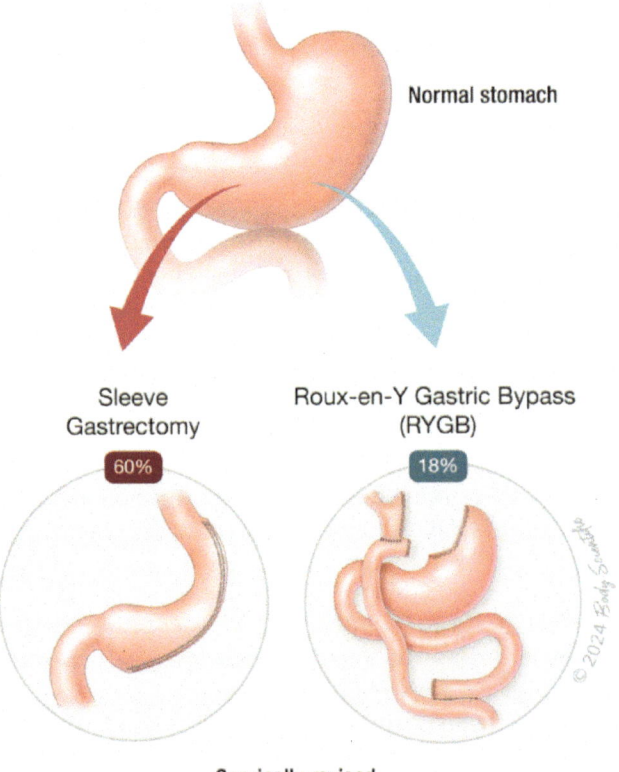

Common Bariatric Procedures*

Normal stomach

Sleeve Gastrectomy
60%

Roux-en-Y Gastric Bypass (RYGB)
18%

Surgically revised

*Less Common –
Duodenal Switch (DS) and Adjustable Gastric Lapband
(due in part, to higher complication rate).

American Society for Metabolic and Bariatric Surgery. (2019). Metabolic and bariatric surgery.

Sleeve Gastrectomy

Vertical sleeve gastrectomy involves removing 85–90% of the stomach. During the procedure, a small tool called a bougie is inserted into the throat and guided down the stomach's inner curve. Surgeons then use a cutting stapler to remove part of the stomach, leaving behind a narrow, sleeve-like portion. This surgery aids in weight loss by limiting the amount of food the stomach can hold and lowering levels of ghrelin, a hormone that increases hunger. Patients can expect to lose about 60% of their excess body weight, with most weight loss occurring within the first year. However, there is a risk of developing GERD, with studies reporting rates of 20–30%. Although the procedure is generally safe, there is a small risk of complications such as bleeding, infection, or vitamin deficiencies, although these occur infrequently.

Roux-en-Y Gastric Bypass

Roux-en-Y gastric bypass is both a restrictive and malabsorptive procedure, meaning it limits the amount of food patients can eat and reduces how many nutrients the body absorbs. During the surgery, a small stomach pouch is created using surgical staples, separating it from the rest of the stomach. The intestines are then rerouted, with the small intestine connected directly to the pouch, forming a "Y" shape. This bypasses a portion of the stomach and small intestine, leading to reduced calorie and nutrient absorption, which aids in weight loss. Patients can expect to lose about 70% of their excess body weight, and the procedure is particularly effective for patients who suffer from GERD, as it also serves as an anti-reflux operation. However, patients must regularly monitor their vitamin levels, as the bypass alters the body's ability to absorb essential nutrients such as calcium, iron, and vitamins A, D, E, and K (Sarna & Otterson, 1989).

Duodenal Switch

The duodenal switch combines aspects of sleeve gastrectomy with an intestinal bypass, resulting in greater malabsorption compared to gastric bypass. Although it offers superior weight loss, this approach carries a higher rate of complications. Long-term follow-up studies have shown that duodenal switch patients, particularly those with super obesity, experience better weight loss and metabolic control compared to gastric bypass patients, although they also face increased risks of complications (Möller et al., 2023).

Endoscopic Sleeve Gastroplasty (ESG)

Endoscopic sleeve gastroplasty is a non-surgical, incision-free procedure used for weight loss. During ESG, a device is attached to the end of a gastroscope, which is inserted into the stomach through the throat. Sutures are placed in the stomach to reduce its volume, mimicking the effects of a sleeve gastrectomy without removing any part of the stomach. ESG is less invasive and has fewer adverse events, such as GERD, but studies suggest that laparoscopic sleeve gastrectomy is more effective in terms of weight loss. The choice between the two procedures depends on patient preferences, safety concerns, and long-term sustainability (Nduma et al., 2023).

POST-OPERATIVE CARE AFTER BARIATRIC SURGERY

Post-operative care following bariatric surgery is crucial for ensuring long-term success and minimizing complications. According to the American Society for Metabolic and Bariatric Surgery (ASMBS) 2022 guidelines, comprehensive follow-up care includes regular monitoring of nutritional status, as patients are at risk for deficiencies in vitamins and minerals such as iron, calcium, vitamins D and B12, with lifelong supplementation often required. Special consideration should be given to Black patients, who may face higher rates of complications such as venous thromboembolism (VTE), higher readmission rates, and less overall weight loss post-surgery (Welsh et al., 2020). Ensuring access to culturally competent care, addressing health disparities, and offering tailored support is critical for this population. Adherence to dietary and exercise recommendations, along with psychological support to manage emotional challenges and lifestyle adjustments, is also essential. Regular follow-up appointments help assess progress, monitor for potential complications, and ensure patients maintain long-term health and success after metabolic and bariatric surgery (American Society for Metabolic and Bariatric Surgery, 2022).

COMPLICATIONS OF BARIATRIC SURGERY

A study conducted in 2020, Helah Amirian and colleagues demonstrated that 30 days after bariatric surgery the rate of pulmonary embolism in African American patients nearly doubled compared to their White counterparts (Amirian et al., 2020a). Although VTE is a known risk factor for post-surgical pulmonary embolism, there was little statistical difference in pre-operation VTE between African American and White patients. This raises the question: What aspect of MBS is nearly doubling the risk of pulmonary embolism in African Americans, especially when pre-existing VTE does not appear to be the cause? The answer likely lies in the low inclusion rates of Black people in research studies and sociological determinants of health, such as a lack of resources in disadvantaged neighborhoods, limited access to therapy, and misinformation about health literacy (Johnson et al., 2024).

VTE was the third most common reason for hospital readmission among African American patients who underwent MBS within 30 days. Historically,

VTE research has predominantly included White participants. A 2016 study suggest that specific genetic variations prevalent in the Black population may be independently linked to VTE (Hernandez, 2016). Therefore, healthcare providers should consider these specific genetic markers when assessing VTE risk in Black patients, ensuring more accurate diagnosing and reducing post-operative complications.

In addition to fear of surgical complications, the underutilization of MBS among Black patients is partially due to community-wide views and the stigmatization of both obesity and bariatric surgery. Despite the proven efficacy of surgery, it is often seen as a last resort for those perceived as "beyond help" (Chao et al., 2022). This stigma, combined with cultural perceptions of obesity, prevents many from considering a procedure that could significantly improve their quality of life.

Excess Skin after Bariatric Surgery

Excess skin, also referred to as "redundant skin," is common after bariatric surgery, with over 90% of patients reporting it post-operatively (Sadeghi et al., 2022). Redundant skin can have both physical and psychological effects. Consulting with a plastic surgeon to address this issue can be helpful in improving quality of life. However, body contouring procedures after weight loss are usually not covered by insurance. These procedures may involve multiple areas of the body, such as abdominoplasty (tummy tuck), brachioplasty (upper arm lift), breast lifts, and thigh lifts. It is important to wait until weight has stabilized before undergoing body contouring, as further weight loss afterward can negatively affect the results (Cabbabe, 2016).

In general, patients who undergo body contouring after MBS tend to have better long-term outcomes in maintaining a lower BMI compared to those who do not. Additionally, it eliminates intertrigo (a skin condition caused by friction), improves comfort, and enhances overall self-confidence. Although 96% of patients who undergo gastric bypass surgery will experience loose skin, body contouring is typically not covered by insurance, meaning patients must pay out of pocket for these procedures. On average, patients who receive body contouring surgery after MBS have an annual income of $71,000 (Rhemtulla et al., 2019). In low-income populations, life-enhancing procedures like abdominoplasty and liposuction post-MBS become unaffordable and inaccessible, contributing to ongoing health inequities.

RACIAL AND ETHNIC DISPARITIES IN BARIATRIC SURGERY

Despite the widespread success of bariatric surgeries, it is crucial to recognize that outcomes vary significantly across racial and ethnic groups. Research shows that Black patients are more likely to experience complications within the first 30 days after surgery compared to White patients, although rates of serious complications and mortality remain similar (Amirian et al., 2020). Studies also show that Black patients tend to experience less weight reduction post-surgery. The reasons for this disparity are unclear, but contributing factors may include differences in post-operative care, healthcare access, insurance coverage, and cultural perceptions of weight and health.

These disparities highlight the need for healthcare systems to adopt more culturally sensitive approaches to care. Addressing barriers such as limited access to health insurance and the underrepresentation of Black patients in weight loss surgery can help close the gap in outcomes. Equally important is building trust with minority communities by providing personalized care that respects their cultural beliefs and values, ensuring healthcare equity for all.

While challenges remain, MBS is a powerful and effective tool in addressing obesity across all populations. Black patients, in particular, experience significant health improvements, including better management of conditions like diabetes and hypertension. Notably, despite differences in weight loss outcomes, Black patients have a lower risk of reoperation compared to White patients, demonstrating the overall effectiveness of the procedure. By prioritizing equity and cultural competency in healthcare, we can create pathways for more individuals to benefit from these life-changing interventions, fostering healthier, more empowered futures for everyone.

FROM STATISTICS TO SOLUTIONS IN METABOLIC AND BARIATRIC SURGERY

There are several evidence-based approaches to reducing the barriers Black patients face in accessing and benefiting from bariatric surgery:

- **Provider Education and Training:** Culturally sensitive care begins with the education of healthcare providers. Research shows that implicit bias and lack of cultural competency can affect the quality of care Black patients receive. Implementing mandatory cultural competence training for bariatric surgeons and healthcare teams is essential. This training should focus on addressing weight bias, understanding the cultural stigmas surrounding obesity, and improving patient–provider communication. Increasing the number of Black surgeons can also improve the likelihood of culturally competent care.

- **Community Outreach and Education:** Community-based programs that educate Black communities about the benefits and safety of MBS could help reduce the stigma surrounding the procedure. These programs should involve trusted healthcare professionals who can provide culturally relevant information. Empowering patients with knowledge fosters more informed decision-making about surgical interventions.

- **Increasing Access through Policy Reform:** Insurance coverage and accessibility remain significant barriers for many Black patients. Policies should be reformed to reduce the financial burden of MBS by expanding Medicaid and Medicare coverage, particularly for post-surgery body contouring procedures, which are often inaccessible to lower-income patients. This would reduce complications related to redundant skin and improve long-term outcomes.

- **Multidisciplinary Care Teams:** Multidisciplinary care teams, including nutritionists, psychologists, and social workers, can provide comprehensive support to Black patients undergoing bariatric surgery. These teams can help address psychological barriers to surgery, such as internalized stigma, while ensuring patients have the nutritional and emotional support needed to succeed post-surgery.

- **Tailored Pre- and Post-Operative Care:** Given the higher rates of complications and reduced weight loss among Black patients, tailored pre- and post-operative care is essential. Monitoring for venous thromboembolism (VTE) risk in Black patients should include testing for genetic variations specific to this population to ensure accurate diagnoses and reduce post-operative complications. Post-surgery care should also include personalized strategies to address nutrient absorption and weight loss challenges specific to Black patients, including tailored nutrition and physical activity plans.

- **Patient Advocacy and Support Networks:** Establishing patient advocacy groups and support networks focused on the Black community can provide emotional and psychological support. These groups can also serve as a bridge between patients and healthcare providers, ensuring patients feel empowered to seek care. Peer support groups, where Black patients who have undergone MBS share their experiences, can help reduce fear and stigma. One example of an online bariatric support group is ObesityHelp.com.

COSMETIC PROCEDURES: LIPOSUCTION AND NON-SURGICAL FAT REDUCTION

Many people mistakenly believe that procedures like liposuction and non-surgical fat reduction are designed to treat obesity, but this is not the case. These techniques are primarily used for cosmetic purposes, aiming to contour the body by eliminating areas of excess fat that don't respond well to diet or exercise. These methods have become increasingly popular, including within the Black community, as they offer customized solutions for body enhancement without addressing medical conditions such as obesity.

LIPOSUCTION: A SURGICAL OPTION FOR FAT REMOVAL

Liposuction is a common surgical procedure that targets and removes fat deposits in specific areas such as the abdomen, thighs, and arms. This procedure involves the use of a small tube, called a cannula, to physically extract fat from the body, resulting in a more contoured appearance. One of the key benefits of liposuction is the immediate and noticeable change in body shape, offering a more dramatic effect than non-surgical options. However, patients must take into account that recovery can take several weeks, during which compression garments may be needed to minimize swelling and support the healing process. Like all surgeries, there are risks, including the possibility of infection, bleeding, or complications related to anesthesia. Despite these considerations, liposuction remains a top choice for those seeking long-term body reshaping (Bartow & Raggio, 2023).

NON-SURGICAL FAT REDUCTION TECHNIQUES

Non-surgical methods for fat reduction have gained popularity as less invasive alternatives to liposuction. These techniques include options such as fat-freezing (cryolipolysis), ultrasound treatments, and procedures that use radiofrequency or lasers to reduce fat. Cryolipolysis, for example, involves cooling fat cells to the point where they break down, while ultrasound and radiofrequency methods use energy to disrupt fat cells. One of the main advantages of non-surgical options is the minimal downtime, allowing individuals to return to normal activities soon after treatment. However, these procedures typically yield more gradual and modest fat reduction compared to liposuction and often require multiple sessions to achieve the desired result. Studies suggest that, on average, non-invasive treatments can reduce fat thickness by about 2 cm (Mulholland et al., 2016). These techniques are effective for mild to moderate fat reduction, but they are generally not suitable for those seeking more substantial results.

CONCLUSION

In conclusion, metabolic and bariatric surgery (MBS) offers significant benefits for individuals struggling with obesity and related comorbidities, leading to meaningful improvements in weight, health, and quality of life.

This chapter has provided an in-depth look at the effectiveness of common procedures such as sleeve gastrectomy and Roux-en-Y gastric bypass, while also addressing the associated risks, including nutritional deficiencies and GERD. Additionally, the chapter emphasizes the cosmetic impacts of weight loss, including excess skin, and highlights the potential role of body contouring surgeries in patient care. The discussion also underscored the racial and ethnic disparities present in MBS outcomes, particularly among Black patients, who face higher complication rates and reduced weight loss. These disparities highlight the critical need for more equitable healthcare practices, culturally sensitive care, and policy reforms to improve access and outcomes for all populations. Ultimately, MBS is a powerful tool in the fight against obesity, but achieving optimal results requires a multifaceted approach that addresses both clinical and social factors.

CLINICAL CONSIDERATIONS CHECKLIST: BARIATRIC SURGERY CHALLENGES AND BENEFITS

Here's a seven-question conversation guide that patients and doctors can use during an office visit to discuss bariatric surgery, based on the information in this chapter.

1. What are the benefits of bariatric surgery for my specific health conditions, such as diabetes or hypertension?

2. What are the different types of bariatric surgery, and which one would be the best option for me?

3. What are the potential risks and complications, including those that may be more common in Black patients?

4. How can we address post-surgery challenges such as excess skin or nutrient deficiencies?

5. What are the insurance requirements for bariatric surgery, and how can we navigate any barriers specific to my coverage?

6. What kind of lifestyle changes will I need to make both before and after surgery to ensure long-term success?

7. What support will be available to me, including psychological and community resources, to help me through this process?

Chapter 13

Pediatric Obesity in the Black Community

Kathi Earles, MD, MPH, DABOM,
Dannielle A. Brown, MD, and
Tiffani Bell-Washington, MD, MPH, MBA, FAPA, FOMA,
DABOM, DABLM

> Childhood obesity isn't some simple, discrete issue. There's no one cause we can pinpoint. There's no one program we can fund to make it go away. Rather, it's an issue that touches on every aspect of how we live and how we work.
>
> —Michelle Obama

PREVALENCE

Mirroring the trend in the Black adult population, obesity in Black children is more prevalent than in White children in both sexes and at every age of development. Obesity in children is defined using percentiles to account for growth throughout the various ages and stages of development. Class 1 obesity in childhood is defined as a BMI of >95 percentile for age and sex. Class 2 and class 3 obesity are defined as a BMI >120% and >140 percentile, respectively. Although a deceleration of obesity occurred in children 6 and younger between 2017–2018, the rate continued to increase in Black adolescents. Currently, the prevalence of obesity in Black children is 35.2% compared to 28.5% in White children and is higher for each sex and every age group in Black youth (Ogden et al., 2018). Additionally, in children older than 6 years of age, the prevalence increases as the child ages for both Black and White communities; however, the prevalence in Black youth remains significantly greater. If the current trend continues, more than 57% of children ages 2–19 years will have obesity in 2050. Studies have demonstrated that these racial/ethnic disparities begin early during the prenatal period and remain throughout adulthood (Taveras et al., 2010). Associated with the rise in obesity in Black children is the rise in associated comorbidities, including the early development of type 2 diabetes, hypertension, and metabolic dysfunction-associated steatohepatitis. The origin of obesity in this young population is multifactorial and includes the interplay between genetics, environment, sleep, behavior, stress, and additional features impacting the

    DOI: 10.1201/9781032622217-16

postnatal period. Additionally, many of the attributes within the built environment, including the lack of green space and access to healthy food, contribute to the higher prevalence of obesity in Black children.

ETIOLOGY

Genetics

Historically, understanding the association of genetics to obesity in the Black community was hampered by studies with patients predominantly of European descent and an insufficient representation of patients of African descent. The absence of a representative sample of patients of African ancestry in earlier studies made the comparison less than accurate. Early genomic-wide association studies with predominantly White patients identified an association between the FTO gene (fat mass and obesity-related gene) located on chromosome 16 and obesity. However, a similar association in people of African descent was as evident (Grant et al., 2008). Unlike the earlier studies, which lacked a representative sample of patients of African descent, a study performed at the University of Illinois in Black adults concluded that the FTO gene in Black patients was in fact associated with obesity (Chalazan et al., 2021). Furthermore, the genomic-wide association studies included in The African Ancestry Genetics Consortium (AAAGC) identified the variant responsible for gene expression in subcutaneous and visceral adipose tissue (Agrawal et al., 2022). Successive research on obesity in the pediatrics population has identified that heritability in BMI ranges between 40–70% (Hebebrand et al., 2003).

In addition to the role of genetics, epigenetics—defined as heritable changes in gene expression without changes in the DNA sequence—contribute to the development of obesity (Mahmoud, 2022). The impact of epigenetics contributes to the increase in obesity through several generations. The most common mechanism of epigenetic modification seen throughout the genome is DNA methylation/demethylation (Tirthani et al., 2023). Fetal programming refers to the in utero period when the maternal diet impacts the health of the fetus (Van Dijk et al., 2015). Maternal undernutrition and subsequent intrauterine growth retardation contribute to alterations in fetal insulin metabolism. Although viewed as a survival mechanism in utero, ensuing exposure of offspring to a nutrient-rich and high-caloric environment can lead to the development of obesity. The process in which the fetus adapts in utero to a nutrient-poor environment and later develops obesity when exposed to a high-caloric milieu is known as the thrifty gene hypothesis (Mandy & Nyirenda, 2018). Additionally, maternal undernutrition has been linked to the development of fetal obesity. Maternal diabetes, low pre-pregnancy weight, and younger maternal age are all maternal factors that are associated with future development of obesity in childhood (Lawlor et al.,

2012). Maternal exposure to toxins, including polycyclic aromatic hydrocarbons, cigarette smoke, and organochlorides, can result in epigenetic modifications. In addition to maternally derived epigenetic contributions, paternal overnutrition, low-protein diet, and pre-diabetes have been linked to epigenetic factors resulting in obesity in the developing child. Other epigenetic factors associated with obesity in both children and adults include a high intake of fried foods, sugary beverages, saturated fats, sleep disturbances, and a sedentary lifestyle (Heianza & Qi, 2017).

Polygenetic inheritance implies that a trait is controlled by two or more genes; however, the phenotypic expression of the genes are dependent upon additional predisposing circumstances. Polygenetic effects of obesity compose a larger proportion of obesity causes compared to monogenic causes. Purely genetic causes of obesity typically present early in life prior to 5 years of age with hyperphagia, severe obesity, and distinctive characteristics unique to each type.

Table 13.1 Monogenetic Syndromes Associated with Obesity

Genetic Syndromes Associated with Obesity	Traits	Comments
MC4R Deficiency	>Linear growth, body mass, insulin levels, + decreased blood pressure	
POMC Deficiency	>Growth during childhood, >ACTH, mild hypothyroidism, red hair, pale skin in Caucasian children	
Leptin Deficiency	Normal linear growth in childhood with deceleration during adulthood, hypothalamic dysfunction, rapid development of obesity, altered immune system	Responsive to Leptin treatment
Leptin Receptor Deficiency	Normal linear growth in childhood with deceleration during adulthood, hypothalamic dysfunction, rapid development of obesity, altered immune system	Non-responsive to Leptin treatment
Alstrom Deficiency	Insulin resistance, T2DM, short stature, visual and hearing impairment, cardiomyopathy, hearing failure, hepatic dysfunction	

(Continued)

Table 13.1 (Continued)

Genetic Syndromes Associated with Obesity	Traits	Comments
Bardet–Biedl Syndrome	Normal height, polydactyly, hypogonadism, renal malformation, polyuria, polydipsia, retinal dystrophy, cognitive impairment	
Brain-Derived Neurotrophic Factor Deficiency	Hyperphagia, hyperactivity, learning disability, impaired short-term disability	Wilms tumor-aniridia BDNF associated with a subset of deletions located on 11p.12
Albright's Hereditary Osteodystrophy	Round face, short stature, brachydactyly, subcutaneous ossifications, + mild developmental delay	Maternal inheritance is associated with pseudohypoparathyroidism type 1a
Beckwith–Wiedemann Syndrome	Macroglossia, macrosomia, hemi hyperplasia, visceromegaly, anterior wall defects, visceromegaly, neonatal hypoglycemia, embryonal tumors, renal anomalies	Genetic modification in chromosome 11p1.5
Cohen Syndrome	Intellectual disability, hypotonia, prominent upper teeth, retinal dystrophy, broad nasal tip, smooth and shortened philtrum, thick hair and eyebrows, long eyelashes, microcephaly, joint hyperextensibility	Alteration in chromosome 11p15.5
Prader–Willi Syndrome	Almond-shaped eyes, long narrow head, triangular mouth, small hands and feet, underdeveloped genitals, poor feeding and hypotonia in infancy, later development of temper tantrum, hyperphagia	

Source: Data extracted from Kaur et al. (2017).

Additional contributors to the early development of obesity include gestational age at birth and parental obesity and stress. Maternal nutritional status and pre-pregnancy weight have been implicated in contributing to the weight of the newborn. Specifically, maternal pregnancy overweight and obesity are associated with babies who are large for gestational age. Regarding the role of gestational age, preterm infants have a greater likelihood of developing childhood obesity, although the cause remains unclear (Gnawali, 2021). Parental obesity is a strong predictor of obesity, extending throughout the life of the offspring, and is more closely associated to maternal pre-pregnancy and excessive maternal weight gain during pregnancy than to paternal obesity. Gestational diabetes and macrosomia are both complications linked to maternal obesity and increase the prevalence of obesity and type 2 diabetes in the offspring (Shakya et al., 2015). It has been postulated that potential mechanisms for the association between gestational obesity and macrosomia are influenced by several factors, including the impact of maternal insulin resistance. Maternal insulin resistance and hyperglycemia appear to influence excessive fetal growth, macrosomia, and increased adiposity (Catalano, 2010). The impact of maternal obesity has been illustrated in metabolic and bariatric studies demonstrating that offspring born prior to the bariatric procedure have a significantly higher prevalence of obesity compared to offspring born to the same mother after the procedure. Maternal obesity more than doubles the development of obesity in the child compared to the additive effect of paternal obesity (Isganaitis et al., 2017). Although this is true, the risk increases to a greater extent when both parents have obesity (Lima et al., 2021). In addition to the impact of parental obesity, toxic stresses experienced by the fetus in utero, including those due to familial poverty and maternal stress, have been connected to the initiation of metabolic and neuroendocrine adaptations, resulting in biologic phenotypes and the development of obesogenic behaviors.

Family Interactions and Home Environment

Parental modeling of eating behavior and family habits have been linked to dietary practices and weight of the offspring (Mahmoud, 2022). Quantities and types of food in the home influence food preferences and eating behavior of the offspring.

Home environmental attributes have demonstrated an impact on healthy eating and activity, including home organizational practices, consumption of sugary beverages, portion size, snacking, screen time, sedentary behavior, sleep practices, smoke exposure, and psychosocial stress. A review of 32 studies demonstrated that greater organization of the home environment, including partaking in meals as a family unit, are inversely proportional to obesity. This finding was noted for both younger and older children.

The presence of sugary sweetened beverages was found to be associated with obesity in the vast majority of studies. This finding also demonstrated a link between sugary sweetened beverages and dental and medical diseases, which precipitated the American Academy of Pediatrics (AAP) publication of a policy statement calling for policies restricting the consumption of these beverages in children and adolescents (Muth et al., 2019).

Although additional studies noting the long-term impact of consuming large amounts of ultra-processed high-caloric snack foods including fast food and junk food are needed, initial studies noted a positive correlation with fat deposition and body weight (Costa et al., 2020). Subsequent studies are needed to investigate the long-term impact on cognitive function and long-term growth and development.

Studies investigating the impact of eating outside of the home have demonstrated higher fat and larger portion sizes compared to food eaten within the home and as a family (Cohen & Bhatia, 2012). Eating out has been associated with consuming larger portion sizes and higher calories, but eating at home as a family has been associated with a lower risk of developing obesity during childhood (Devilal et al., 2023).

Screen Time

A multitude of studies have demonstrated the impact of increased screen time on increasing BMI in children and adults. Tripathi and others have shown a dose-response impact on the development of childhood adiposity demonstrating that more than 2 hours of screen time per day is positively associated with a larger risk of overweight or obesity (Tirthani et al., 2023). Additionally, the type of food consumed is of low to no nutritional value and frequently high in fat, sugar, and salt content. A study by Tahir and others reported the risk of developing obesity or becoming overweight increases by 42% with more than 2 hours of television per day (Tahir et al., 2019). Stationary time spent on other devices, including tablets, mobile phones, computers, game consoles, accessing the internet, video games, social media, and a variety of apps, increases sedentary time and contributing to the development of obesity. Another contributing feature is the preponderance of advertisements focused upon fast foods and beverages. Studies have demonstrated that viewing advertisements for fast foods, snacks, and beverages has a positive impact on consuming larger quantities of high-caloric food with little nutritional value (American Psychological Association, 2010).

Quantity of Sleep

Numerous studies have demonstrated the inverse relationship between sleep quantity and obesity in the pediatric population (Miller et al., 2015). Studies have also demonstrated that children 13 years old or younger with less than 10 hours of sleep have an increased risk of obesity by 76%. Historical trends on the quantity of sleep time have demonstrated a decline by 75 minutes per night per year. As sleep duration has decreased, the inverse has occurred regarding the prevalence of obesity in the pediatric population (Hart et al., 2013). Reasons for the impact of decreased sleep on adiposity are still unfolding, but one known mode of action is the alterations in satiety and hunger hormones, resulting in an increase in caloric intake and decreased energy expenditure (Balagopal et al., 2010).

Smoke Exposure

Studies have demonstrated the impact of smoke exposure beginning in utero. Specifically, the impact of maternal tobacco smoke has been linked to increased BMI of offspring when compared to infants without exposure. The ramifications of in utero exposure appear to be long lasting, as evidenced by an increase in waist circumference, BMI, and central and abdominal fat distribution, which extend into adulthood (Albers et al., 2018). Additionally, exposure beginning in childhood up to age 8 years demonstrated higher BMIs than in non-exposed children (Mourino et al., 2022). When investigating the impact of secondhand smoke on children ages 12–15 years from low- to middle-income neighborhoods, a study demonstrated an increased prevalence of obesity (Koyanagi et al., 2020).

Psychosocial Stress

Maternal stress impacts the endocrine system throughout the life of the child. A study by Tate and others demonstrated that psychological stress experienced by the fetus has been linked to a higher risk of childhood obesity continuing throughout adolescence (Tate et al., 2015). Additionally, other in utero and childhood toxic stresses including poverty have been implicated in the development of metabolic maladaptation, resulting in obesogenic behaviors and biological phenotypes (O'Connor, 2017). Stress experienced throughout childhood has been linked to defective coping skills, including eating in the absence of hunger, decreased physical activity, depression, and sleep disruption (Rojo et al., 2021). Weight stigma, teasing, and bullying experienced throughout childhood have also been linked to binge eating, decreased activity, social isolation, avoidance of medical care, and poor mental health (Gmeiner & Warschburger, 2023).

Increased adverse childhood experiences (ACEs), including neglect, caregiver mental illness, substance use, economic insecurity, physical, emotional, or sexual abuse, domestic violence, or loss of a parent due to death or incarceration, appear to double the risk of both overweight and obesity when compared to children without a history of repeated ACEs (Burke et al., 2011).

Postnatal Contributors

Early breastfeeding cessation and antibiotic use have been implicated in contributing to pediatric obesity. Several studies have demonstrated that breastfed babies are better able to regulate their energy intake, resulting in a lower risk of obesity compared to bottle-fed infants (Taveras et al., 2010).

The association is more robust when breastfeeding is continued throughout the first year of life compared to cessation at or before 6 months of age (Azad et al., 2018).

Feeding practices including over-concentrated formula, high-protein formulas, adding cereal to the bottle, introduction of complementary foods prior to 4 months of age, and placing infants in the bed with a bottle have all been linked to an elevated BMI later in childhood. Additionally, children who have rapid weight gain during the first 2 years of life are 3.5 times more likely to develop overweight and obesity later in life (Zheng et al., 2018).

Although the impact of early antibiotic use prior to age 2 years appears to be mixed, the association between repeated antibiotic use prior to age six months, including the use of broad-spectrum antibiotics and subsequent overweight and obesity, is stronger. Potential contributors are an early alteration of the gut microbiota altering the microbiome.

Childhood risk factors, including medical and developmental issues, can also contribute to excess weight gain. Some associated contributors are endocrine disorders, special healthcare needs impacting nutrition and physical activity, ADHD, and weight-promoting drugs.

Endocrine disorders are implicated in less than 1% of all causes of pediatric obesity and may be associated with either endogenous or exogenous glucocorticoid excess. Growth failure or short stature with an abnormally high BMI have been associated with growth hormone deficiency, pseudohypoparathyroidism type 1a, and hypothyroidism (Halilagic & Moschonis, 2021).

Children with Special Needs

Children with special needs such as developmental delay, physical disabilities, and autism spectrum disorder face unique challenges that contribute to weight gain and obesity. Physical activity limitations may impact children with developmental disabilities, resulting in a more sedentary lifestyle that promotes weight gain. Feeding challenges, including selective eating habits or emotional eating, may result in an increase in caloric intake. Additionally, several medications used to manage the symptoms of specific conditions such as autism spectrum disorder may increase appetite and subsequent weight gain.

Social Determinants of Health

Social determinants of health (SDOH) that adversely contribute to the prevalence of obesity in marginalized Black communities are environmental and physical conditions such as a lack of adequate and safe recreational space, proximity to food deserts, limited access to nutritious foods, economic disparities, substandard education, and exposure to chronic stress. Studies indicate that the impact of economic instability during childhood

Table 13.2 Special Considerations Regarding Obesity in Children with Special Healthcare Needs

Condition	Prevalence	Association to Weight Gain	Physical Features	Mental Features	Etiology	Evidence-Based Treatment
Developmental Disabilities	1 in 6	• Reduced physical activity • Feeding difficulty	• Delayed growth, motor and muscle tone impairments	• Cognitive impairments, difficulty in self-regulation, emotional and developmental delay	• Genetic and prenatal factors resulting in reduced physical activity and difficulty feeding	• Multidisciplinary approach Physical therapy • Occupational therapy • Nutrition counseling • Behavioral intervention
Physical Disabilities	Variable	• Decreased muscle tone • Limited physical activity	• Muscle weakness, mobility issues, spasticity	• Learning disabilities • Emotional regulation challenges	• Brain injury • Prenatal/postnatal complications	• Adaptive physical therapy • Caloric adaptation • Dietary modification • Speech/feeding therapy
Autism Spectrum Disorder	1 in 36 children	• Food selectivity • Preference for high-calorie, low-nutrient food	• Sensory issues • Feeding difficulties	• Anxiety • Food selectivity • Repetitive behaviors	• Multifactorial • Genetic • Environmental	• Structured feeding programs • Sensory integration • Applied Behavioral Analysis • Occupational therapy
Myelomeningocele	3.4 per 10,000 live births	• Reduced mobility, resulting in lower energy expenditure	• Paralysis below spinal defect • Bowl/bladder issues	• Learning difficulties • Emotional regulation challenges	• Neural tube defect during fetal development	• Physical therapy • Specialized diet • Surgical intervention

(Continued)

Table 13.2 (Continued)

Condition	Prevalence	Association to Weight Gain	Physical Features	Mental Features	Etiology	Evidence-Based Treatment
Attention Deficit Hyperactivity Disorder	5–10% globally	• Impulsive eating behavior	• No overt physical features	• Hyperactivity • Impulsivity • Emotional dysregulation	• Genetic predisposition • Neurotransmitter imbalances	• Behavior therapy • Structured physical activity • Stimulant medication • Counseling
Weight-Promoting Appetitive Traits	1:5 in developed countries	• Predisposition for increased appetite • Lower sensitivity to satiety signals	• Elevate BMI • Excessive appetite	• Impulsivity • Emotional eating • Reduced hunger control	• Genetic predisposition • Environmental influences	• Dietary counseling • Cognitive behavioral therapy • Appetite control interventions • Structured mealtime planning

Sources: Minihan et al. (2007); Bandini et al. (2005).

has an enduring impact on overweight and obesity in adulthood, even when there is an upward economic trend following early childhood (Sturm, 2014). Parental educational attainment also impacts the prevalence of obesity in their offspring. In a study by Buoncristiano and others, more than 5,000 children ages 6–9 years old whose parents had a lower level of education also had a higher prevalence of obesity when compared to children whose parents had a higher level of education (Music Milanovic et al., 2021). The lasting ramifications of a dysfunctional environment emphasize the necessity for policies that not only address the root causes but also implement comprehensive changes that promote health equity for all children.

PEDIATRIC OBESITY: FUNDAMENTALS OF OBESITY TREATMENT

Early intervention and comprehensive management are essential to prevent obesity-related complications and promote lifelong health. Effective treatment strategies emphasize a family-centered approach, which involves engaging parents and caregivers in creating a supportive home environment that encourages healthy eating, regular physical activity, and limited screen time. A multidisciplinary team consisting of pediatricians, dietitians, behavioral specialists, and physical activity experts is crucial to addressing all aspects of a child's health, ensuring that interventions are tailored to meet the unique needs of each patient (Yu et al., 2021).

In addition to addressing contributing SDOH, components of pediatric obesity management include Medical Nutrition Therapy (MNT), behavioral interventions, and age-appropriate physical activity recommendations. Medical nutrition guided by a registered dietitian focuses on improving dietary quality by incorporating nutrient-dense foods while remaining mindful of cultural preferences and socioeconomic barriers (Fitzpatrick & Wischenka, 2020). Behavioral interventions, such as motivational interviewing and cognitive-behavioral therapy (CBT), help address underlying psychological factors, including emotional eating, body image concerns, and low self-esteem. Interventions should be culturally sensitive and adapted to their specific needs to enhance engagement and adherence (Taveras et al., 2015).

Pharmacotherapy and bariatric surgery are considered for adolescents with obesity and comorbid conditions, especially when lifestyle modifications alone are insufficient. Long-term follow-up and maintenance are essential to ensure continued progress and prevent weight regain. Regular check-ins, family support, and community resources can all contribute to sustaining healthy habits over time and improving health outcomes for children and adolescents (Gruber & Haldeman, 2009).

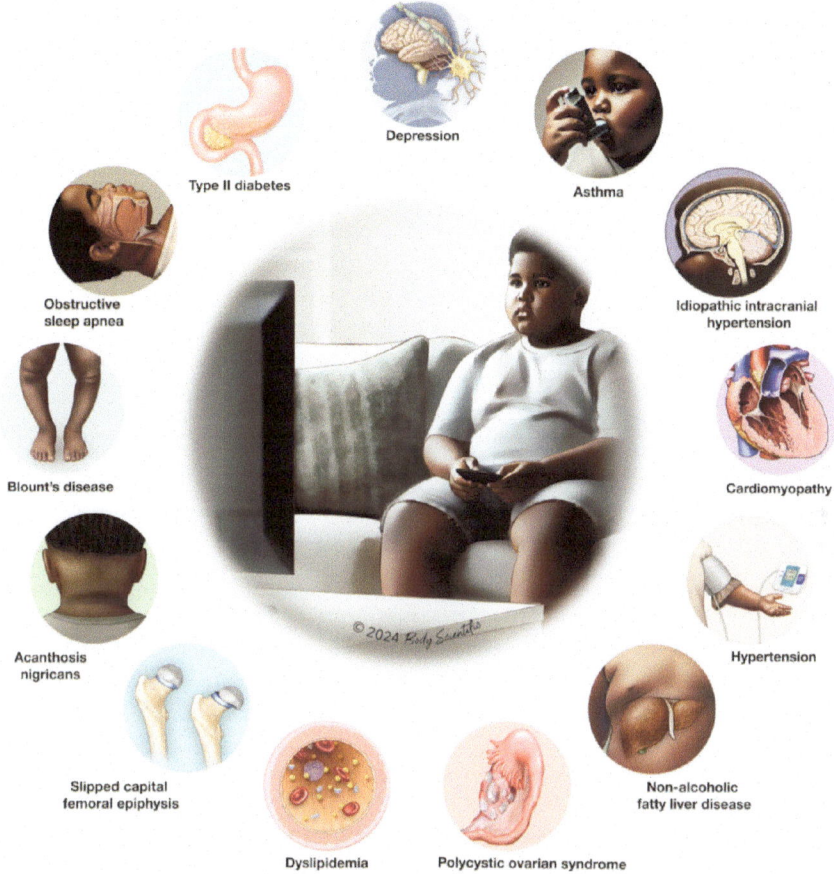

Comorbidities in Childhood Obesity

Depression

Type II diabetes

Asthma

Obstructive sleep apnea

Idiopathic intracranial hypertension

Blount's disease

Cardiomyopathy

Acanthosis nigricans

Hypertension

Slipped capital femoral epiphysis

Non-alcoholic fatty liver disease

Dyslipidemia

Polycystic ovarian syndrome

© 2024 Body Scientific

Table 13.3 Key Components of Pediatric Obesity

Component	Key Considerations
Family-Centered Care	• Involves parents, caregivers, and extended family in supporting healthy behaviors at home and recognizing the importance of family influence in Black communities. • Build family support by incorporating cultural values and traditions, structure meal times, limit screen time, and use community resources.
Multidisciplinary Approach	• Team includes culturally competent pediatricians, dietitians, behavioral specialists, community health workers, and physical activity experts. • Ensure coordinated, culturally competent care targeting all aspects of the child's health and incorporate trusted community voices in planning and implementation.

(Continued)

Table 13.3 Key Components of Pediatric Obesity (Continued)

Component	Key Considerations
Medical Nutrition Therapy (MNT)	• Focus on improving dietary quality by incorporating nutrient-dense and culturally relevant foods while educating on potential healthy modifications to traditional recipes. • Consider cultural food preferences, barriers such as food deserts, limited access to affordable healthy foods, and socioeconomic constraints.
Physical Activity Recommendations	• Children and adolescents should engage in 60 minutes of physical activity daily, incorporating community sports, dance classes, or neighborhood-based activities. • Promote activities rooted in community traditions, such as double Dutch, neighborhood sports, or dance. Consider safety, access to recreational spaces, and socioeconomic constraints.
Behavioral Interventions	• Address psychological factors such as body image, emotional eating, and impacts of racism and stigma through culturally sensitive CBT and motivational interviewing. • Focus on culturally sensitive strategies to address systemic racism and weight stigma. Integrate interventions that address historical mistrust of healthcare systems and promote resilience and self-esteem.
Pharmacotherapy	• Consider for adolescents with severe obesity when lifestyle interventions alone are insufficient. Assure equitable access and monitoring for side effects. • Assess and address mistrust in medical system and facilitate equitable access to pharmacological intervention.
Metabolic and Bariatric Surgery	• Reserved for severe cases with comorbidities and performed in specialized centers with a focus on addressing potential disparities in surgical access and outcomes. • Conducted by an experienced multidisciplinary team with attention to equity in outcomes, culturally competent communication, and comprehensive follow-up support.
Long-Term Follow-Up	• Continuous support through regular check-ins, monitoring, community resources, and faith-based and culturally relevant support systems to prevent weight regain and sustain healthy habits. • Incorporate community-based organizations, faith leaders, culturally resonant mentors, and trusted community voices to ensure long-term success while addressing potential barriers to maintaining healthy behaviors.

LIFESTYLE MEDICINE-BASED MODIFICATIONS FOR BLACK CHILDREN WITH OVERWEIGHT AND OBESITY

Family-Centered Lifestyle Modifications

Family-centered care continues to be a cornerstone of pediatric obesity management. Engaging parents and caregivers in the child's weight management plan ensures that the entire family adopts healthy behaviors, creating a supportive environment that fosters long-term success.

Recent findings suggest that traditional parenting styles—authoritative, authoritarian, permissive, and uninvolved—each have a different impact on a child's dietary habits and weight status. Parenting styles that balance a high level of responsiveness, structure, and encourage a positive attitude, such as authoritative styles, have been shown to promote healthier eating habits and may offer protection against increased BMI and assist in shaping long-term healthy behaviors (Kiefner-Burmeister & Hinman, 2020).

To Implement Effective Family-Based Interventions

1. **Model Healthy Eating Behaviors:** Parents should demonstrate healthy eating behaviors, such as choosing nutrient-dense foods and controlling portion sizes, and involve children in meal planning and preparation.
2. **Use Positive Reinforcement:** Reinforce healthy eating and physical activity with praise and rewards that are non-food related.
3. **Create Structured Family Meals:** Regular family meals, characterized by set meal times and healthy food choices, have been shown to improve dietary habits and lower the risk of obesity (Bailey-Davis et al., 2019).

Culturally Appropriate Dietary Modifications for Black Children with Obesity: Guidance for Parents and Clinicians

Promoting healthy eating in Black communities requires a deep understanding of cultural food traditions, family dynamics, and existing barriers such as food insecurity. Culturally tailored dietary modifications should maintain the essence of traditional dishes while enhancing their nutritional value. For Black children with obesity, it's important to make dietary changes that feel inclusive and respectful of their cultural identity.

Key Advice for Parents

1. **Use Healthier Cooking Techniques for Traditional Dishes**
   - Encourage the use of healthier cooking methods like baking, grilling, or steaming traditional dishes. For example, instead of frying

chicken, consider oven-baking it with a seasoned, whole-wheat crust.
- Modify recipes for family favorites by substituting lard or butter with heart-healthy oils such as olive oil or avocado oil.
- Use herbs and spices like thyme, rosemary, garlic, and cayenne pepper to add flavor without relying on high-sodium seasonings like ham hocks or bouillon cubes. Consider using smoked turkey or a dash of liquid smoke for that traditional flavor in greens.

2. **Incorporate More Plant-Based Ingredients**
   - Introduce more plant-based proteins like beans, lentils, and black-eyed peas in meals. These foods are not only culturally familiar but also packed with fiber and nutrients.
   - Experiment with adding more leafy greens such as kale, mustard greens, and collard greens, prepared in a way that reduces added fats and retains their natural flavors.

3. **Adjust Portion Sizes and Balance Plates**
   - Educate children and families on creating balanced plates using the "MyPlate" method, adapted to include culturally relevant food items. A balanced plate should have a smaller portion of meat, a larger portion of vegetables, a whole grain, and a small serving of healthy fat.
   - Use smaller plates and bowls to control portion sizes and encourage slow eating practices that allow children to recognize fullness cues.

4. **Preserve Cultural Identity through Food**
   - Help families create "heritage plates" by emphasizing the nutritional benefits of traditional foods that are part of the African Diaspora, such as okra, yams, and millet.
   - Encourage parents to involve children in meal preparation to pass down healthy versions of family recipes, making it a learning experience that preserves family traditions.

5. **Be Mindful of Family Food Rules and Traditions**
   - Respect and engage in conversations about family food rules and routines. For example, if there is a tradition of Sunday family dinners, help parents make this a time to reinforce healthier food choices through shared family meals that emphasize fruits, vegetables, and lean proteins.

Key Advice for Clinicians

1. **Provide Culturally Sensitive Nutrition Education**
   - When providing nutritional advice, frame suggestions within the context of foods familiar to Black families. For instance, suggest

using lower-sodium seasonings in collard greens or sweet potatoes prepared with less added sugar.

- Use visuals and examples that reflect the cultural context of your patients. For instance, show images of modified soul food dishes and provide recipes that reduce sugar, salt, and unhealthy fats without compromising flavor.

2. **Address Food Insecurity and Accessibility**
   - Understand that many Black families face barriers to accessing fresh produce and healthy foods due to living in food deserts. Importantly, lack of access is not equal to lack of desire to be healthy; therefore, we must be careful not to pass judgment on intent or ability to follow recommendations.
   - Consider connecting families to resources such as community gardens, food pantries, or mobile farmer's markets that serve under-resourced areas.
   - Work with local grocers and faith-based organizations to create programs that promote the availability and affordability of fresh, healthy options.

3. **Engage Community Resources and Cultural Leaders**
   - Partner with local community leaders, churches, and Black-owned businesses to provide nutrition workshops and cooking demonstrations that highlight healthy versions of traditional recipes.
   - Encourage the use of community kitchens or cooking classes that teach families how to prepare familiar dishes in healthier ways, making the experience collaborative and engaging.

4. **Address Health and Socioeconomic Barriers with Sensitivity**
   - Avoid a prescriptive approach that feels judgmental or dismissive of cultural preferences. Understand that food is deeply tied to identity, social status, and tradition in Black communities.
   - Be mindful of economic barriers when suggesting dietary changes. If recommending fresh produce, consider discussing how to buy affordable frozen or canned options without added sugars or salts.

5. **Highlight the Historical and Cultural Significance of Certain Foods**
   - Recognize and discuss the historical significance of some foods that may be perceived as "unhealthy." For example, certain high-calorie or nutrient-dense foods may have roots in survival strategies developed during times of economic hardship or limited access to fresh produce.
   - Use this historical context to suggest *small, manageable changes* rather than completely eliminating cherished foods. This approach can help families feel respected and valued, making them more receptive to change.

Physical Activity and Active Play for Black Children

Physical activity recommendations should focus on incorporating culturally relevant and accessible activities that resonate with Black children and their families. Community-based strategies, such as using local recreation centers or organizing neighborhood sports events, can increase adherence and long-term engagement.

Research suggests that effective parenting strategies, such as modeling physical activity and establishing clear expectations, significantly influence children's levels of physical activity (Vega-Diaz et al., 2023). This suggests that family involvement is crucial for increasing activity levels and improving long-term health outcomes. Additionally, fathers' involvement in physical activity is an emerging area of focus, demonstrating that parental roles need to be diversified in interventions (Latomme et al., 2023).

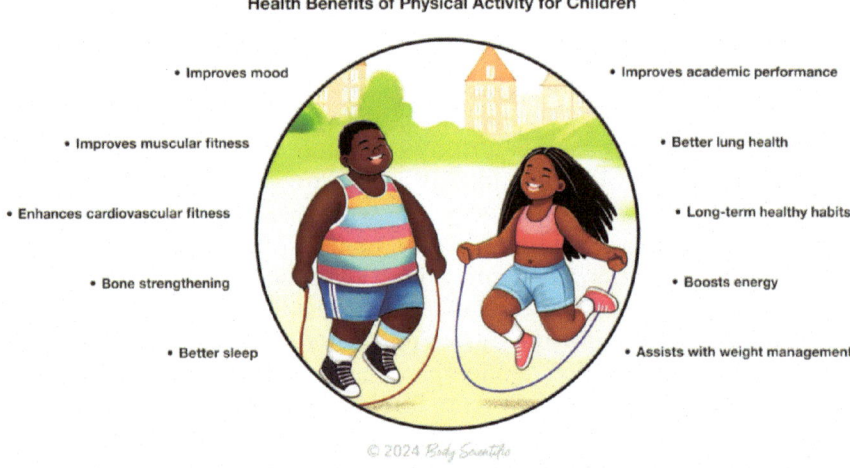

Health Benefits of Physical Activity for Children

• Improves mood
• Improves muscular fitness
• Enhances cardiovascular fitness
• Bone strengthening
• Better sleep

• Improves academic performance
• Better lung health
• Long-term healthy habits
• Boosts energy
• Assists with weight management

© 2024 *Body Scientific*

U.S. Department of Health and Human Services.
Physical Activity Guidelines for Americans, 2nd edition.
Washington, DC: U.S. Department of Health and Human Services; 2018.

Updated Recommendations

1. **Encourage Family-Based Physical Activities**: Activities such as family walks, dance sessions, or community sports events increase engagement and reinforce positive physical activity habits.
2. **Incorporate Community Resources**: Utilize schools, community centers, and faith-based organizations to promote regular physical activity in a safe and structured environment.
3. **Address Barriers to Physical Activity**: Consider neighborhood safety, accessibility, and cultural preferences when developing physical activity plans for families.

Behavioral Strategies to Address Emotional Eating and Body Image

Behavioral strategies should focus on the psychological aspects of obesity and emphasize positive coping mechanisms to reduce emotional eating and body dissatisfaction. Incorporating mindfulness-based practices and resilience training can help children develop a positive body image and healthier relationships with food.

Recent literature highlights the effectiveness of the Obesity Parenting Intervention (OPTION) Scale, which measures parental influences on child eating behaviors and obesity-related practices (Figueroa et al., 2019). The OPTION Scale provides a validated tool for assessing and guiding behavioral interventions in diverse communities.

Behavioral Strategies

1. **Implement the OPTION Scale:** Use this scale to identify specific parental practices that contribute to obesity risk and to tailor interventions that support healthier eating behaviors.
2. **Focus on Mindful Eating Practices:** Teach children and families to recognize hunger and fullness cues, avoid distractions during meals, and create a calm eating environment.
3. **Address Weight-Related Stigma:** Conduct family sessions to reduce weight-related stigma and promote body positivity and self-acceptance.

Long-Term Maintenance and Follow-Up Strategies

Long-term follow-up is essential for maintaining progress and preventing weight regain. Research conducted during COVID-19 emphasizes the need for structured follow-up plans that include not only clinical visits but also community-based support and digital tools for tracking behavior and outcomes (Mantena & Keshavjee, 2021).

Long-Term Strategies

1. **Integrate Community Support Networks:** Partner with community-based organizations and schools to create sustainable support networks.
2. **Use Digital Health Tools:** Employ digital apps or telehealth platforms to maintain engagement between visits.
3. **Focus on Empowerment and Self-Efficacy:** Reinforce the child's and family's capacity to manage health behaviors independently.

COMORBIDITIES OF CHILDHOOD OBESITY

The disease of obesity is associated with numerous comorbidities that impact the quality of life through associated comorbidities. The abundance of comorbidities affect almost every organ in the body, including the skin, gastrointestinal tract, renal, musculoskeletal, psychological, dental, cardio-vascular, respiratory, and endocrine system. The most commonly reported comorbidities associated with obesity are hypertension, metabolic syndrome, and dyslipidemia. Several of these comorbidities require special consideration in children, including type 2 diabetes, polycystic ovarian syndrome (PCOS), and cancer.

The greater prevalence of type 2 diabetes in Black adults reflects the continuation of obesity and type 2 diabetes in the Black children. Consistent with the prevalence of obesity in Black compared to White children, the prevalence of type 2 diabetes is also greater in Black children compared to White children. The SEARCH for Diabetes in Youth Population Study found that 6% of White children ages 10–19 years old were diagnosed with type 2 diabetes compared to 33% of Black children within the same age range (Hamman et al., 2014). An interesting feature associated with the increased prevalence of type 2 diabetes in Black children is that White children have significantly more visceral fat after adjusting for total body fat. Black children, however, are more insulin resistant independent of visceral fat accumulation and location (Allister-Price, 2005 [2019]). This is believed to be a contributing feature to the increased prevalence of type 2 diabetes in Black children even when comparing with similar weight in White children.

Polycystic ovarian disease (PCOS) is seen in females of childbearing ages and is associated with enlarged and dysfunctional ovaries, insulin resistance, and excess androgen (Trent & Gordon, 2020). Although the increased frequency of gonadotropin-releasing hormone and high ratio of luteinizing hormone to follicle-stimulating hormone have been identified as the underlying cause, the exact etiology is not well understood. While obesity plays a role in the development of PCOS, oxidative stress, epigenetics, environmental toxins, insulin resistance, hyperandrogenism, and diet appear to contribute to development of the disease (Sadeghi et al., 2019). In addition to PCOS being a comorbidity of obesity, it also increases other obesity-related comorbidities, including type 2 diabetes, metabolic syndrome, cardiovascular disease, anxiety, and depression.

An alarming number of studies have demonstrated a clear association between obesity throughout the pediatric period and several types of cancer, including colorectal, endometrial, ovarian, thyroid, and pancreatic cancer (Mohammadian Khonsari et al., 2023).

A review of the literature conducted by Weihe and others showed a significant association between childhood and adolescent obesity and the overall incidence of malignancies (Weihe et al., 2020). Another review indicated an incremental increase in ovarian cancer based upon the BMI and early-onset obesity and a significantly greater risk of adult colorectal cancer. Obesity is therefore a modifiable risk for cancer (Mohammadian Khonsari et al., 2023).

Table 13.4 Comorbidities Associated with Childhood Obesity

Organ	Comorbidity
Skin	• Acanthosis nigricans • Psoriasis
Gastrointestinal	• Metabolic dysfunction • Micronutrient deficiencies • Associated fatty liver disease • Constipation • Gastroesophageal Reflux
Renal	• Glomerulosclerosis • Enuresis
Musculoskeletal	• Pain • Acute injuries • Impaired balance and coordination • Impaired muscle strength • Gait disturbances • Postural malalignment • Fractures • Slipped capital epiphysis • Blount's disease
Psychosocial	• Reduced self-esteem • Depression • Anxiety • Disordered eating • Body dissatisfaction
Dental	• Cavities • Periodontal disease
Cardiovascular	• Hypertension • Dyslipidemia • Endothelial dysfunction • Left ventricular hypertrophy
Respiratory	• Asthma • Obstructive sleep apnea • Impaired exercise tolerance • Sleep disorders • Poorer outcomes with viral infections • Hypoventilation syndrome
Endocrine	• Impaired glucose tolerance • Polycystic ovarian syndrome • Delayed or accelerated puberty • Metabolic syndrome • Type 2 diabetes
Cancer	• Colorectal, leukemia, Hodgkin's disease, colorectal, postmenopausal breast, uterine, esophageal, kidney, and pancreatic cancers

Source: Table created by author from information from Kumar and Kelly (2017).

OBESOGENIC PRESCRIPTION MEDICATIONS

A modifiable contributor to overweight and obesity are commonly prescribed medications that promote weight gain in the pediatric population. Some allergy and asthma medications have been linked to weight gain in pediatrics. Of note, the highest prevalence of asthma in children in the United States is also the group that has the highest prevalence of obesity in the pediatric community. In the United States, Black and Brown children have higher rates of asthma and its complications when compared with White children. Additionally, frequently prescribed medications associated with obesity include certain antiepileptics, antidepressants, antipsychotics, anxiolytics, migraine therapy, mood stabilizers, and psychostimulants. Many of the commonly prescribed medications known to contribute to the disease of obesity have alternative products with less of an impact on weight gain.

Table 13.5 Obesogenic Medications

	Obesogenic Medication	Non-Obesogenic Medication
Allergy and Asthma	• Antihistamines • Systemic steroids	• Inhaled nasal steroid • Montelukast
Antidepressants	• Amitriptyline • Sertraline • Nortriptyline • Paroxetine	• Bupropion • Imipramine HCL • Citalopram • Fluoxetine • Buspirone
Antiepileptics	• Carbamazepine • Gabapentin • Valproate	• Felbamate • Lamotrigine • Phenytoin • Topiramate
Antipsychotics	• Clozapine • Haloperidol • Mirtazapine • Risperidone • Quetiapine	• Molindone • Pimozide
Anxiolytics	• N/A	• Alprazolam • Lorazepam
Migraine Therapy	• Amitriptyline • Atenolol • Gabapentin • Imipramine • Nortriptyline • Propranolol	• Lamotrigine • Topiramate • Zonisamide
Psychostimulant	• N/A	• Amphetamine • Methylphenidate • Dextroamphetamine sulfate

Source: Table created by author from information extracted from Hales et al. (2022).

Table 13.6 Evaluation and Treatment of Pediatric Obesity

Evaluation Component	Key Points	Special Considerations and Relevant Points
HISTORY		
Past Medical History	• Prenatal risk factors • Presence of comorbid conditions • Growth trajectory over time (abrupt vs. chronic weight gain) • Developmental milestones • Past interventions for weight management • Medication history	• Consider identifying early-onset obesity (<5 years) as it may indicate genetic factors or syndromic obesity. • Investigate prenatal exposures, including maternal weight gain, gestational diabetes, and smoking, which are linked to higher obesity risk in offspring. • Medication history should emphasize medications known to cause weight gain (e.g., antipsychotics, corticosteroids).
Family History	• Potential genetic susceptibilities • Obesity-related comorbidities	• Include a three-generation family history to assess for familial patterns of obesity and metabolic syndrome. • Consider genetic counseling for syndromic obesity when indicated.
Social History	• Living arrangements • Family structure • Cultural values • Recent life stressors • School environment • Peer relationships • History of bullying • Mental and emotional well-being • Socioeconomic factors	• Be sensitive to social determinants of health that may affect the ability to implement lifestyle changes (e.g., safe areas for exercise, access to healthy foods). • Bullying or weight stigma can significantly impact mental health and should be screened for routinely.
Nutrition History	• Food preferences (home meals vs. fast food) • Eating patterns • Frequency of snacks • Frequency of sugary beverages • Portion sizes • Attitude toward food	• Assess for emotional eating patterns or using food as a coping mechanism. • Consider referral to a dietitian or nutritionist for detailed dietary assessment. • Use age-appropriate visual aids to gauge portion sizes in younger children.

(Continued)

Table 13.6 Evaluation and Treatment of Pediatric Obesity (Continued)

Evaluation Component	Key Points	Special Considerations and Relevant Points
Physical Activity	• Frequency, type, duration of exercise • Participation in organized sports or other group activities • Access to safe spaces • Screen time • Sleep patterns	• Calculate total screen time and identify sedentary behaviors, including use of mobile devices and gaming consoles. • Sleep disturbances can contribute to obesity and should be routinely evaluated.
PHYSICAL EXAM		
Vital Signs	• Blood pressure—assess for hypertension • Heart rate and respiratory rate—assess for tachycardia, tachypnea	• Consider using age-specific blood pressure percentiles for accurate assessment. • Evaluate for orthostatic changes, which may indicate dehydration or other comorbidities.
Growth Patterns	• Measure height and weight—assess growth percentiles • Track growth trends over time—changes in height velocity, changes in weight gain	• Use BMI percentiles for age and gender, rather than absolute BMI values, to diagnose overweight and obesity in children. • Evaluate for rapid weight gain or loss, which can indicate underlying metabolic or endocrine disorders.
HEENT	• Papilledema • Tonsillar hypertrophy • Dental caries • Goiter	• Papilledema may indicate increased intracranial pressure, often linked with severe obesity and pseudotumor cerebri. • Assess for obstructive sleep apnea risk in children with tonsillar hypertrophy.
GI	• Hepatomegaly	• Hepatomegaly may indicate non-alcoholic fatty liver disease (NAFLD), which is highly prevalent in obese children. • Further evaluation with liver ultrasound or liver function tests may be warranted.

(Continued)

Table 13.6 (Continued)

Evaluation Component	Key Points	Special Considerations and Relevant Points
Cardiopulmonary	• Dyspnea • Rales	• Consider a sleep study if obesity hypoventilation syndrome or obstructive sleep apnea is suspected. • Evaluate for asthma, as it often coexists with obesity and can be worsened by excess weight.
MSK (Musculoskeletal)	• Gait abnormalities • Joint pain • Decreased range of motion • Genu varum or valgum • Pes planus	• Assess for signs of Blount's disease or slipped capital femoral epiphysis (SCFE) in children with severe obesity and leg pain. • Refer to orthopedics if significant joint deformities or pain are present.
Skin	• Acanthosis nigricans • Intertrigo • Hirsutism • Acne • Striae	• Acanthosis nigricans is a clinical marker of insulin resistance. • Intertrigo (skin fold inflammation) is common in obesity and may require topical treatment.
LABORATORY EVALUATION		
Evaluate for Insulin Resistance/Diabetes	• Fasting blood glucose • Hgb A1c	• Consider an oral glucose tolerance test (OGTT) if diabetes is suspected but not confirmed with initial labs.
Evaluate for Dyslipidemia	• Fasting lipid profile	• Early identification of dyslipidemia is crucial, given its long-term cardiovascular risks. Repeat annually in children with elevated BMI.
Evaluate for Liver Disease/Hepatic Steatosis	• Liver function tests (particularly ALT)	• Elevated ALT levels warrant further imaging and assessment for NAFLD. • Lifestyle modification is the first-line treatment for NAFLD.
Evaluate to Rule Out Hypothyroidism	• Thyroid function tests	• Thyroid disease should be ruled out, especially in the presence of growth delay, fatigue, or poor weight management.

(Continued)

Table 13.6 Evaluation and Treatment of Pediatric Obesity (*Continued*)

Evaluation Component	Key Points	Special Considerations and Relevant Points
Other Tests to Consider	• Complete blood count • Basic metabolic panel • Vitamin D level	• Vitamin D deficiency is common in pediatric obesity and should be corrected if present. • Consider other micronutrient deficiencies (e.g., iron, B12) if dietary intake is poor.

Source: Kumar and Kelly (2017). American Academy of Pediatrics, AAP section on Obesity, AAP Committee on Nutrition, AAP American Heart Association. Public policy to reduce sugar. *Pediatrics.*

CONCLUSION

Pediatric obesity is a multifaceted condition with far-reaching implications for physical and mental health. When obesity begins in childhood, it often leads to the early development of comorbidities typically seen in adults, such as type 2 diabetes, hypertension, and cardiovascular disease. Longitudinal studies have shown that approximately 55% of children with obesity continue the trajectory into adulthood, with 80% of adolescents with obesity becoming adults with obesity (Drozdz et al., 2021). Early onset of obesity increases the risk for premature mortality and severe health complications in adulthood, emphasizing the critical need for early intervention.

The Harvard Growth study revealed that being overweight in adolescence is a strong predictor of numerous adverse health outcomes in adulthood independent of adult weight, including hypertension, hyperinsulinemia, and elevated lipid levels (Must et al., 2012). This highlights the critical need to address obesity during childhood to prevent severe comorbidities and improve long-term health outcomes, particularly in Black children, who experience a disproportionately higher prevalence of obesity and its related complications (Obita & Alkhatib, 2022).

Effectively managing pediatric obesity requires a culturally sensitive, family-centered approach that respects the child's environment, family dynamics, and cultural background. Clinicians must prioritize strategies that involve the entire family, integrate community resources, and address broader systemic factors contributing to health inequities, such as food deserts and limited access to safe spaces for physical activity. Understanding these variables is essential to developing impactful clinical interventions and implementing public health policies that promote equitable healthcare and sustainable health outcomes.

Table 13.7 Approved Pharmacotherapy for Pediatric Obesity

Anti-Obesity Medication	Administration	Mode of Action	Weight Loss	Dose	Common Side Effects	Contraindications
Orlistat	• 12 ≥ years • Approved for long-term use	• Inhibits gastric and pancreatic lipase • Reversibly inactivates ≤ 91.4% enzymes • Decreases fat absorption	5%	• 120 oral mg TID before meals	• Flatulence • Steatorrhea • Fecal urgency	• Pregnancy • Breastfeeding • Cholestasis • Chronic malabsorption syndrome • Known hypersensitivity • Increased urinary oxalate • Severe liver injury • Hypothyroidism • Cholelithiasis following substantial weight loss • Co-administration with cyclosporine not recommended • Should not co-administer antiepileptics and antiretrovirals • Take fat-soluble vitamins

(Continued)

Table 13.7 Approved Pharmacotherapy for Pediatric Obesity (Continued)

Anti-Obesity Medication	Administration	Mode of Action	Weight Loss	Dose	Common Side Effects	Contraindications
Liraglutide 3 mg	• ≥ Use with reduced-calorie diet and increased PE • ≥ 12 years BW > 60 kg initial BMI ≥30 kg/m²	• Stimulates POMC • Promotes satiety	5.8%	• Dose escalation • 0.6 mg × 1 wk • 1.2 mg × 1 wk • 1.8 mg × 1 wk • 2.4 mg × 1 wk	• Nausea • Diarrhea • Constipation • Vomiting • Injection site reaction • Headache • Hypoglycemia in type 2 DM • Dyspepsia • Fatigue • Dizziness • Abdominal pain • Inc. lipase • Upper abdominal pain	• Personal or family history of medullary thyroid carcinoma or MEN syndrome type 2 • Known hypersensitivity • Pregnancy
Semaglutide 2.4 mg	• ≥ Use with reduced-calorie diet and increased PE • ≥ 12 years BW > 60 kg initial BMI ≥30 kg/m²	• Stimulates POMC • Promotes satiety	16%	• Dose escalation • 0.25 mg × 1 month • 1.2 mg × 1 month • 1.8 mg × 1 month • 2.4 mg × 1 month	• As above	• Personal or family Hx of medullary thyroid carcinoma or MEN syndrome 2 • Known hypersensitivity • Pregnancy
Phentermine/ Topiramate	• ≥ 12 years and older with BMI at 95th percentile or greater for age and sex	• Phentermine increases firing of POMC • Topiramate inhibits stimulation of NPY		• Dose escalation • 3.75 mg/23 mg × 2 wks • Maintenance 7.5 mg/46 mg • May increase to 11.25 mg/69 mg × 2 wks • 15 mg/92 mg	• Paresthesia • Dizziness, dysgeusia • Insomnia • Constipation • Dry mouth	• Pregnancy • Glaucoma • Hyperthyroidism • Concomitant use of MAOIs • Hypersensitivity or idiosyncrasy to sympathomimetic amines

Source: Created by authors from data from Kühnen et al. (2022).

CLINICAL CONSIDERATIONS CHECKLIST: PEDIATRIC OBESITY

Pediatric obesity is a multifactorial condition requiring a comprehensive approach that considers genetic, behavioral, environmental, and cultural factors. When managing pediatric obesity in Black children, it is crucial to apply a culturally sensitive approach that respects family values and addresses potential socioeconomic barriers. This clinical considerations section aims to provide healthcare professionals with evidence-based strategies and culturally appropriate guidance for assessing, treating, and supporting children with obesity.

1. **Family-Centered Assessment and Interventions**
   - Include the family in all aspects of obesity management. Family dynamics, parenting styles, and home environment significantly influence a child's weight and dietary habits. Use family-based counseling to improve overall health behaviors (Kiefner-Burmeister & Hinman, 2020).
   - Engage parents in modeling healthy behaviors and encourage shared physical activities. Empower families to establish structured mealtimes and make healthy food choices.

2. **Culturally Appropriate Nutritional Modifications**
   - Adapt traditional recipes to healthier versions while maintaining cultural relevance. Highlight the nutritional benefits of heritage foods such as okra, sweet potatoes, and beans, using cooking methods like steaming or grilling instead of frying.
   - Address food insecurity by connecting families to community resources such as local farmer's markets, faith-based organizations, or grocery programs that offer fresh produce and healthy options at lower costs.

3. **Screening for Social Determinants of Health (SDOH)**
   - Assess the impact of SDOH such as access to safe recreational spaces, food deserts, and parental education levels on health outcomes. Recognize that economic instability and unsafe environments may limit opportunities for physical activity and healthy eating.

4. **Behavioral Health and Emotional Support**
   - Evaluate for weight-related stigma, bullying, and mental health conditions such as anxiety or depression, which can contribute to unhealthy coping mechanisms like emotional eating. Use validated tools, such as the Pediatric Symptom Checklist, to screen for emotional and behavioral concerns.

- Incorporate mindfulness-based interventions and resilience training to support positive body image and reduce emotional eating.

5. **Physical Activity Recommendations**
   - Promote culturally relevant and community-based physical activities, such as local sports clubs or dance classes that resonate with the child's interests.
   - Encourage active play in safe spaces and collaborate with community leaders to create structured physical activities when neighborhood safety is a concern.

6. **Long-Term Maintenance and Follow-Up**
   - Develop structured follow-up plans that incorporate community support, telehealth, and digital tools for tracking behaviors and outcomes. Encourage regular follow-up visits to address potential weight regain and reinforce positive lifestyle habits.

7. **Consideration of Genetic and Epigenetic Factors**
   - Be aware of genetic predispositions to obesity, such as FTO and MC4R gene variations more commonly identified in Black populations. Include a family history of early-onset obesity and metabolic conditions to guide tailored interventions (Fitzpatrick & Wischenka, 2020).

PRE-VISIT QUESTIONNAIRE FOR PEDIATRIC OBESITY ASSESSMENT

Providing families with a pre-visit questionnaire allows clinicians to gather comprehensive information to tailor obesity interventions more effectively. The following questions are designed to help identify lifestyle patterns, dietary behaviors, and psychosocial factors contributing to weight gain:

1. What is your child's typical eating schedule?
   (Include meals, snacks, and beverages.)

2. How often does your child consume fast food or sugary beverages (e.g., soda, sweet tea, fruit juices)?

3. Describe your child's physical activity.
   (How often, what type of activities, and for how long?)

4. Does your child have any sleep issues (difficulty falling asleep, staying asleep, or getting up in the morning)?

5. How much screen time does your child typically get each day? (Include television, video games, tablets, and mobile phones.)

6. Have you noticed any patterns of eating in response to stress, sadness, or boredom?
(If yes, provide examples.)

7. What types of foods are most commonly available in your household? (Include staple foods, snack options, and beverages.)

8. Does your child experience teasing, bullying, or negative comments about their weight?
(If yes, how do they respond or cope?)

9. Have there been any recent changes in your family structure, such as a move, new school, or significant stressors?

10. What are your family's main goals for your child's health and weight?

REFERENCES FOR CLINICIANS

Kiefner-Burmeister, A., & Hinman, N. (2020). The role of general parenting style in child diet and obesity risk. Current Nutrition Reports, 9(1), 14–30. https://doi.org/10.1007/s13668-020-00301-9

Ramuscak, N., Shamah-Levy, T., Habib-Mourd, M., Karssen, L., & Nezami, N. et al. (2023). Cross-cutting environmental policies to promote the availability and consumption of sustainable and affordable foods. Frontiers in Public Health, 11, 944648. https://doi.org/10.3389/fpubh.2023.944648

U.S. Department of Agriculture and U.S. Department of Health and Human Services. (2020). Dietary guidelines for Americans, 2020–2025. Dietary Guidelines for Americans. http://DietaryGuidelines.gov

Engberg, E., Leppänen, M. H., Sarkkola, C., & Viljakainen, H. (2021). Physical activity among preadolescents modifies the long-term association between sedentary time spent using digital media and the increased risk of being overweight. Journal of Physical Activity & Health, 18(9), 1105–1112. https://doi.org/10.1123/jpah.2021–0163

References

Agrawal, S., Wang, M., Klarqvist, M. D. R., et al. (2022). Inherited basis of visceral, abdominal subcutaneous and gluteofemoral fat depots. Nature Communications, 13, 3771. https://doi.org/10.1038/s41467-022-30931-2.

Agyemang, P., & Powell-Wiley, T. M. (2013). Obesity and Black women: Special considerations related to genesis and therapeutic approaches. Current Cardiovascular Risk Reports, 7(5), 378–386. https://doi.org/10.1007/s12170-013-0328-7.

Ainsworth, B. E., Haskell, W. L., Herrmann, S. D., Meckes, N., Bassett, D. R. Jr., Tudor-Locke, C., Greer, J. L., Vezina, J., Whitt-Glover, M. C., & Leon, A. S. (2011, August). Compendium of physical activities: A second update of codes and MET values. Medicine & Science in Sports & Exercise, 43(8), 1575–1581. https://doi.org/10.1249/MSS.0b013e31821ece12. PMID: 21681120.

Albers, L., Sobotzki, C., Kuß, O., Ajslev, T., Batista, R. F., Bettiol, H., Brabin, B., Buka, S. L., Cardoso, V. C., Clifton, V. L., Devereux, G., Gilman, S. E., Grzeskowiak, L. E., Heinrich, J., Hummel, S., Jacobsen, G. W., Jones, G., Koshy, G., Morgen, C. S., Oken, E., Paus, T., Pausova, Z., Rifas-Shiman, S. L., Sharma, A. J., da Silva, A. A., Sørensen, T. I., Thiering, E., Turner, S., Vik, T., & von Kries, R. (2018, July). Maternal smoking during pregnancy and offspring overweight: Is there a dose-response relationship? An individual patient data meta-analysis. International Journal of Obesity (London), 42(7), 1249–1264. https://doi.org/10.1038/s41366-018-0050-0. Epub 2018 February 28. PMID: 29717267; PMCID: PMC6685293.

Alhasan, D. M., Riley, N. M., Jackson II, W. B., & Jackson, C. L. (2023). Food insecurity and sleep health by race/ethnicity in the United States. Journal of Nutritional Science, 12, e59. https://doi.org/10.1017/jns.2023.18. PMID: 37252683; PMCID: PMC10214135.

Alick, C. L., Samuel-Hodge, C., Ammerman, A., Ellis, K. R., Rini, C., & Tate, D. F. (2023, February). Motivating weight loss among black adults in relationships: Recommendations for weight loss interventions. Health Education & Behavior, 50(1), 97–106. https://doi.org/10.1177/10901981221129182. Epub 2022 Oct 15. PMID: 36245237; PMCID: PMC9902993.

Allister-Price, C., Craig, C. M., Spielman, D., Cushman, S. S., & McLaughlin, T. L. (2005 [2019]). Metabolic markers, regional adiposity, and adipose cell size: Relationship to insulin resistance in African-American as compared with Caucasian women. International Journal of Obesity, 43(6), 1164–1173. https://doi.org/10.1038/s41366-018-0191-1.

American College of Lifestyle Medicine. (2021). What is lifestyle medicine? https://www.lifestylemedicine.org.

American Medical Association. (2019). H-440.842 Obesity as a disease. AMA Policy Finder. https://policysearch.ama-assn.org/policyfinder/detail/obesity?uri=%2FAMADoc%2FHOD.xml-0-3858.xml.

American Psychological Association. (2010, November 17). The impact of food advertising on childhood obesity. https://www.apa.org/topics/obesity/food-advertising-children.

American Society for Metabolic and Bariatric Surgery. (2022a). 2022 ASMBS and IFSO indications for metabolic and bariatric surgery. https://asmbs.org/resources/2022-asmbs-and-ifso-indications-for-metabolic-and-bariatric-surgery/.

American Society for Metabolic and Bariatric Surgery. (2022b). Estimate of bariatric surgery numbers, 2011–2022. American Society for Metabolic and Bariatric Surgery. https://asmbs.org/resources/estimate-of-bariatric-surgery-numbers/.

Amirian, H., Torquati, A., & Omotosho, P. (2020a). Racial disparity in 30-day outcomes of metabolic and bariatric surgery. Obesity Surgery, 30(3), 1011–1020. https://doi.org/10.1007/s11695-019-04282-9.

Amirian, H., Torquati, A., & Omotosho, P. (2020b). Racial disparities in venous thromboembolism after bariatric surgery: An analysis of the MBSAQIP database. Surgery for Obesity and Related Diseases, 16(8), 1035–1042. https://doi.org/10.1016/j.soard.2020.04.035.

Andreyeva, T., Puhl, R. M., & Brownell, K. D. (2008, May). Changes in perceived weight discrimination among Americans, 1995–1996 through 2004–2006. Obesity (Silver Spring), 16(5), 1129–1134. https://doi.org/10.1038/oby.2008.35. Epub 2008 February 28. PMID: 18356847.

Anekwe, C. V., Jarrell, A. R., Townsend, M. J., Gaudier, G. I., Hiserodt, J. M., & Stanford, F. C. (2020). Socioeconomics of obesity. Current Obesity Reports, 9(3), 272–279. https://doi.org/10.1007/s13679-020-00398-7. PMID: 32627133; PMCID: PMC7484407.

Ard, J. D., Rosati, R., & Oddone, E. Z. (2000, November). Culturally sensitive weight loss program produces significant reduction in weight, blood pressure, and cholesterol in eight weeks. Journal of the National Medical Association, 92(11), 515–523. PMID: 11152083; PMCID: PMC2568323.

Assari, S. (2018). Health disparities due to diminished return among black Americans: Public policy solutions. Social Issues and Policy Review, 12, 112–145. https://doi.org/10.1111/sipr.12042.

Association for Size Diversity and Health (ASDAH). (2024). Health at every size (HAES). https://asdah.org/haes/.

Azad, M. B., Vehling, L., Chan, D., Klopp, A., Nickel, N. C., McGavock, J. M., Becker, A. B., Mandhane, P. J., Turvey, S. E., Moraes, T. J., Taylor, M. S., Lefebvre, D. L., Sears, M. R., Subbarao, P., & CHILD Study Investigators. (2018, October). Infant feeding and weight gain: Separating breast milk from breastfeeding and formula from food. Pediatrics, 142(4), e20181092. https://doi.org/10.1542/peds.2018-1092. PMID: 30249624.

Babatunde, O. A., Bull, E. R., Dombrowski, S. U., McCleary, N., & Johnston, M. (2020). The impact of a randomized dietary and physical activity intervention on chronic inflammation among obese African-American women. Women & Health, 60(7), 792–805. https://doi.org/10.1080/03630242.2020.1777924.

Baicker, K., Cutler, D., & Song, Z. (2010). Workplace wellness programs can generate savings. Health Affairs (Millwood), 29(2), 304–311. https://doi.org/10.1377/hlthaff.2009.0626. Epub 2010 January 14. PMID: 20075081.

Bailey, Z. D., Krieger, N., Agénor, M., Graves, J., Linos, N., & Bassett, M. T. (2017). Structural racism and health inequities in the USA: Evidence and interventions. Lancet, 389, 1453–1463.

Bailey-Davis, L., Kling, S. M. R., Wood, G. C., Cochran, W. J., Mowery, J. W., Savage, J. S., Stametz, R. A., & Welk, G. J. (2019, April 24). Feasibility of enhancing well-child visits with family nutrition and physical activity risk assessment on body mass index. Obesity Science & Practice, 5(3), 220–230. https://doi.org/10.1002/osp4.339. PMID: 31275595; PMCID: PMC6587309.

Bailey-Davis, L., & Savage, J. S. (2023). Editorial: Healthy eating and parenting messages to prevent obesity. Frontiers in Public Health, 11, 1177742. https://doi.org/10.3389/fpubh.2023.

Balagopal, P. B., Gidding, S. S., Buckloh, L. M., Yarandi, H. N., Sylvester, J. E., George, D. E., & Funanage, V. L. (2010, September). Changes in circulating satiety hormones in obese children: A randomized controlled physical activity-based intervention study. Obesity (Silver Spring), 18(9), 1747–1753. https://doi.org/10.1038/oby.2009.498. Epub 2010 January 21. PMID: 20094040.

Bandini, L. G., Curtin, C., Hamad, C., Tybor, D. J., & Must, A. (2005). Prevalence of overweight in children with developmental disorders in the continuous national health and nutrition examination survey (NHANES) 1999–2002. Journal of Pediatrics, 146, 738–743.

Bartow, M. J., & Raggio, B. S. (2023, February 14). Liposuction. In StatPearls [Internet]. Treasure Island, FL: StatPearls Publishing; 2025 January. https://www.ncbi.nlm.nih.gov/books/NBK563135/.

Beach, M. C., Saha, S., & Cooper, L. A. (2006). The Role and Relationship of Cultural Competence and Patient-Centeredness in Health Care Quality. New York: Commonwealth Fund. https://www.commonwealthfund.org/publications/fund-reports/2006/oct/role-and-relationship-cultural-competence-and-patient. Accessed Nov 18, 2019.

Befort, C. A., Thomas, J. L., Daley, C. M., Rhode, P. C., & Ahluwalia, J. S. (2008). Perceptions and beliefs about body size, weight, and weight loss among obese African American women: A qualitative inquiry. Health Education & Behavior, 35(3), 410–426. https://doi.org/10.1177/1090198106290398.

Bell, C. N., Kerr, J., & Young, J. L. (2019). Associations between obesity, obesogenic environments, and structural racism vary by county-level racial composition. International Journal of Environmental Research and Public Health, 16(5), 861. https://doi.org/10.3390/ijerph16050861.

Bischof, G., Bischof, A., & Rumpf, H. J. (2021, February 19). Motivational interviewing: An evidence-based approach for use in medical practice. Deutsches Ärzteblatt International, 118(7), 109–115. https://doi.org/10.3238/arztebl.m2021.0014.

Blasco, B. V., García-Jiménez, J., Bodoano, I., & Gutiérrez-Rojas, L. (2020, August). Obesity and depression: Its prevalence and influence as a prognostic factor: A systematic review. Psychiatry Investigation, 17(8), 715–724. https://doi.org/10.30773/pi.2020.0099. Epub 2020 August 12. PMID: 32777922; PMCID: PMC7449839.

Bleich, S. N., Simon, A. E., & Cooper, L. A. (2012). Impact of patient-doctor race concordance on rates of weight-related counseling in visits by Black and White obese individuals. Obesity (Silver Spring). 20(3), 562–570. https://doi.org/10.1038/oby.2010.330. Epub 2011 January 13. PMID: 21233803; PMCID: PMC3786341.

Brandfon, S., Eylon, A., Khanna, D., & Parmar, M. S. (2023, October 7). Advances in anti-obesity pharmacotherapy: Current treatments, emerging therapies, and challenges. Cureus, 15(10), e46623. https://doi.org/10.7759/cureus.46623. PMID: 37937009; PMCID: PMC10626572.

Brennan, M., & Williams, C. L. (2013). Lifestyle management of cardiovascular risk factors in African American women. ABNF Journal, 24(3), 71–76.

Brown, A., Flint, S. W., & Batterham, R. L. (2022). Pervasiveness, impact and implications of weight stigma. EClinicalMedicine, 47, 101408.

Bryan, C. X. (2024, June 27). What is body inclusivity? Health benefits of body-inclusive fitness. U.S. News & World Report. https://health.usnews.com/wellness/fitness/articles/what-is-body-inclusivity-health-benefits-of-body-inclusive-fitness.

Buchmueller, T. C., Levinson, Z. M., Levy, H. G., Wolfe, B. L. (2016). Effect of the Affordable Care Act on racial and ethnic disparities in health insurance coverage. American Journal of Public Health, 106(8), 1416–1421. https://doi.org/10.2105/AJPH.2016.303155. Epub 2016 May 19. PMID: 27196653; PMCID: PMC4940635.

Burke, N. J., Hellman, J. L., Scott, B. G., Weems, C. F., & Carrion, V. G. (2011, June). The impact of adverse childhood experiences on an urban pediatric population. Child Abuse & Neglect, 35(6), 408–413. https://doi.org/10.1016/j.chiabu.2011.02.006. Epub 2011 June 8. PMID: 21652073; PMCID: PMC3119733.

Byrd, A. S., Toth, A. T., & Stanford, F. C. (2018). Racial disparities in obesity treatment. Current Obesity Reports, 7(2), 130–138. https://doi.org/10.1007/s13679-018-0301-3. PMID: 29616469; PMCID: PMC6066592.

Cabbabe, S. W. (2016, May–June). Plastic surgery after massive weight loss. Missouri Medicine, 113(3), 202–206. PMID: 27443046; PMCID: PMC6140063.

Campbell, K., Foster-Schubert, K., Xiao, L., Alfano, C., Bertram, L. C., Duggan, C., Irwin, M., & McTiernan, A. (2012). Injuries in sedentary individuals enrolled in a 12-month, randomized, controlled, exercise trial. Journal of Physical Activity and Health, 9(2), 198–207. https://doi.org/10.1123/jpah.9.2.198.

Catalano, P. M. (2010, September). Obesity, insulin resistance, and pregnancy outcome. Reproduction, 140(3), 365–371. https://doi.org/10.1530/REP-10-0088. Epub 2010 May 10. PMID: 20457594; PMCID: PMC4179873.

Centers for Disease Control and Prevention (CDC). (2009a). Differences in prevalence of obesity among Black, White, and Hispanic adults—United States, 2006–2008. MMWR, 58(27), 740–744. https://www.cdc.gov/mmwr/preview/mmwrhtml/mm5827a2.htm.

Centers for Disease Control and Prevention (CDC). (2022, December 5). Timeline. U.S. Public Health Service Syphilis Study at Tuskegee. https://www.cdc.gov/tuskegee/timeline.htm.

Chalazan, B., Palm, D., Sridhar, A., Lee, C., Argos, M., Daviglus, M., et al. (2021). Common genetic variants associated with obesity in an African-American and Hispanic/Latino population. PLoS One, 16(5), e0250697. https://doi.org/10.1371/journal.pone.0250697.

Chao, G. F., Diaz, A., Ghaferi, A. A., Dimick, J. B., & Byrnes, M. E. (2022, April). Understanding racially diverse community member views of obesity stigma and bariatric surgery. Obesity Surgery, 32(4), 1216–1226. https://doi.org/10.1007/s11695-022-05928-x. Epub 2022 January 27. PMID: 35088253; PMCID: PMC8794039.

Chatters, L. M., Taylor, H. O., & Taylor, R. J. (2021, September 27). Racism and the life course: Social and health equity for black American older adults. Public Policy Aging Report, 31(4), 113–118. https://doi.org/10.1093/ppar/prab018. PMID: 34691479; PMCID: PMC8528194.

Clapp, B., Ponce, J., Corbett, J., Ghanem, O. M., Kurian, M., Rogers, A. M., Peterson, R. M., LaMasters, T., & English, W. J. (2024). American Society for Metabolic and Bariatric Surgery 2022 estimate of metabolic and bariatric procedures performed in the United States. Surgery for Obesity and Related Diseases, 20(5), 425–431. https://doi.org/10.1016/j.soard.2024.01.012.

Cohen, D. A., & Bhatia, R. (2012). Nutrition standards for away-from-home foods in the USA. Obesity Reviews, 13(7), 618–629.

Cooksey Stowers, K., Jiang, Q., Atoloye, A., Lucan, S., & Gans, K. (2020). Racial differences in perceived food swamp and food desert exposure and disparities in self-reported dietary habits. International Journal of Environmental Research and Public Health, 17(19), 7143. https://doi.org/10.3390/ijerph17197143. PMID: 33003573; PMCID: PMC7579470.

Costa, C., Assunção, M., Loret de Mola, C., Cardoso, J., Matijasevich, A., Barros, A. J. D., & Santos, I. (2020). Role of ultra-processed food in fat mass index between 6 and 11 years of age: A cohort study. International Journal of Epidemiology, 50. https://doi.org/10.1093/ije/dyaa141.

CROWN Coalition. (2024). The CROWN Act. https://www.thecrownact.com/.

Cuevas, A. G., Ong, A. D., Carvalho, K., Ho, T., Chan, S. W. C., Allen, J. D., Chen, R., Rodgers, J., Biba, U., & Williams, D. R. (2020, October). Discrimination and systemic inflammation: A critical review and synthesis. Brain, Behavior, and Immunity, 89, 465–479. https://doi.org/10.1016/j.bbi.2020.07.017. Epub 2020 July 17. PMID: 32688027; PMCID: PMC8362502.

Curry, S. D., and Larkin, C. A. (2002). Social capital, Black social mobility, and health disparities. Annual Review of Public Health, 43, 399–416. https://doi.org/10.1146/annurevpublhealth-05020-112623.

De Souza, A. M. A., Ecelbarger, C. M., & Sandberg, K. (2021). Caloric restriction and cardiovascular health: The good, the bad, and the renin-angiotensin system. Physiology, 36(4), 220–234.

Del Prato, S., Gallwitz, B., Holst, J. J., & Meier, J. J. (2022). The incretin/glucagon system as a target for pharmacotherapy of obesity. Obesity Reviews, 23(2), e13372. https://doi.org/10.1111/obr.13372.

D'Ettorre, G., Pellicani, V., Greco, M., Caroli, A., & Mazzotta, M. (2019). Metabolic syndrome in shift healthcare workers. Med Lavoro, 110(4), 285–292. https://doi.org/10.23749/mdl.v110i4.8350. PMID: 31475690; PMCID: PMC7809991.

Devilal, D., et al. (2023). Cooking and its impact on childhood obesity: Systematic review. Journal of Nutrition Education and Behavior, 55(9), 677–688.

Diez-Roux, A. V., & Mair, C. (2010). Neighborhoods and health. Annals of the New York Academy of Sciences, 1186, 125–145. https://doi.org/10.1111/j.1749-6632.2009.05333.x. PMID: 20201871.

Drozdz, D., Alvarez-Pitti, J., Wójcik, M., Borghi, C., Gabbianelli, R., Mazur, A., Herceg-Čavrak, V., Lopez-Valcarcel, B. G., Brzeziński, M., Lurbe, E., & Wühl, E. (2021). Obesity and cardiometabolic risk factors: From childhood to adulthood. Nutrients, 13(11), 4176. https://doi.org/10.3390/nu13114176.

Duello, T. M., Rivedal, S., Wickland, C., & Weller, A. (2021). Race and genetics versus 'race' in genetics: A systematic review of the use of African ancestry in genetic studies. Evolution, Medicine, and Public Health, 9(1), 2021, 232–245. https://doi.org/10.1093/emph/eoab018.

Earles, K., Ard, J., & Stanford, F. C. (2020, June). A call to action—The need to address obesity in the black community. Journal of the National Medical Association, 112(3), 243–246. https://doi.org/10.1016/j.jnma.2020.03.006. Epub 2020 April 28. PMID: 32354562; PMCID: PMC9908366.

Eden, M. (2023). Quantifying racial discrimination in the 1944 GI Bill. Explorations in Economic History, 90, 101542. https://doi.org/10.1016/j.eeh.2023.101542.

Eskandari, F., Lake, A. A., Rose, K., Butler, M., & O'Malley, C. (2022, August 5). A mixed-method systematic review and meta-analysis of the influences of food environments and food insecurity on obesity in high-income countries. Food Science & Nutrition, 10(11), 3689–3723. https://doi.org/10.1002/fsn3.2969. PMID: 36348796; PMCID: PMC9632201.

Fallon, E. A., Wilcox, S., & Ainsworth, B. E. (2005). Correlates of self-efficacy for physical activity in African American women. Women & Health, 41(3), 47–62.

Figueroa, R., Saltzman, J. A., Aftosmes-Tobio, A., & Davison, K. K. (2019, December). The Obesity Parenting Intervention Scale: Factorial validity and invariance among Head Start parents. American Journal of Preventive Medicine, 57(6), 844–852. https://doi.org/10.1016/j.amepre.2019.08.013. PMID: 31753267; PMCID: PMC8167826.

Finley, R. V. (2023, April 2). Empowering Health Literacy in Making Informed Health Decisions. LinkedIn. https:// www.linkedin.com/pulse/empowering-health-literacy-role-critical-thinking-finley-ph-d.

Fitzpatrick, S. L., & Wischenka, D. M. (2020). Health disparities and pediatric obesity: Influencing factors and intervention strategies. Current Obesity Reports, 9(4), 315–324.

Foster, G. D., Borradaile, K. E., Sanders, M. H., et al. (2009). A randomized study on the effect of weight loss on obstructive sleep apnea among obese patients with type 2 diabetes: The Sleep AHEAD study. Archives of Internal Medicine, 169, 1619.

Frank, L. D., Andresen, M. A., & Schmid, T. L. (2004). Obesity relationships with community design, physical activity, and time spent in cars. American Journal of Preventive Medicine, 27(2), 87–96. https://doi.org/10.1016/j.amepre.2004.04.011. PMID: 15261894.

Fulton, M., Dadana, S., & Srinivasan, V. N. (2023, October 26). Obesity, stigma, and discrimination. In StatPearls [Internet]. Treasure Island, FL: StatPearls Publishing. https://www.ncbi.nlm.nih.gov/books/NBK554571/.

Fung, T. T., van Dam, R. M., Hankinson, S. E., Stampfer, M., Willett, W. C., & Hu, F. B. (2010). Low-carbohydrate diets and all-cause and cause-specific mortality: Two cohort studies. Annals of Internal Medicine, 153(5), 289–298. https://doi.org/10.7326/0003-4819-153-5-201009070-00003. PMID: 20820038; PMCID: PMC2989112.

Gardner, C. D., Trepanowski, J. F., Del Gobbo, L. C., et al. (2018). Effect of low-fat vs low-carbohydrate diet on 12-month weight loss in overweight adults and the association with genotype pattern or insulin secretion: The DIETFITS randomized clinical trial. JAMA, 319, 667.

Garvey, W. T., et al. (2016). American Association of Clinical Endocrinologists and American College of Endocrinology comprehensive clinical practice guidelines for medical care of patients with obesity. Endocrine Practice, 22, 1–203.

George, A., & Guyenet, S. J. (2024). Neurobiology of obesity: Pathways and mechanisms. Endocrine Reviews, 45(3), 309–351. https://doi.org/10.1210/endrev/bnad010.

Ginsburg, B. M., Daley, S. F., & Sheer, A. J. (2024, March 10). Overcoming stigma and bias in obesity management. In StatPearls [Internet]. Treasure Island, FL: StatPearls Publishing. https://www.ncbi.nlm.nih.gov/books/NBK578197/.

Glasgow, R. E., Askew, S., Purcell, P., et al. (2013). Use of RE-AIM to address health inequities: Application in a low-income community health center-based weight loss and hypertension self-management program. Translational Behavioral Medicine, 3(2), 200–210. https://doi.org/10.1007/s13142-013-0191-0.

Gmeiner, M. S., & Warschburger, P. (2023). Interrelation between weight and weight stigma in youth: Is there evidence for an obesogenic vicious cycle? European Child & Adolescent Psychiatry, 32(4), 697–704.

Gnawali, A. (2021, December 19). Prematurity and the risk of development of childhood obesity: Piecing together the pathophysiological puzzle. A literature review. Cureus, 13(12), e20518. https://doi.org/10.7759/cureus.20518. PMID: 35070553; PMCID: PMC8765585.

Goode, R. W., Webster, C. K., & Gwira, R. E. (2022, December). A review of binge-eating disorder in black women: Treatment recommendations and implications for healthcare providers. Current Psychiatry Reports, 24(12), 757–766. https://doi.org/10.1007/s11920-022-01383-8. Epub 2022 November 12. PMID: 36370263; PMCID: PMC9789195.

Gonsahn-Bollie, S. (2021). Embrace You: Your Guide to Transform Weight Loss Misconceptions into Lifelong Wellness. Publish Your Gift.

Gothe, N. P., & Kendall, B. J. (2016, November 16). Barriers, motivations, and preferences for physical activity among female African American older adults. Journal of Gerontology & Geriatric Medicine, 2, 2333721416677399. https://doi.org/10.1177/2333721416677399. PMID: 28138500; PMCID: PMC5117257.

Grandner, M. A., Williams, N. J., Knutson, K. L., Roberts, D., & Jean-Louis, G. (2016, February). Sleep disparity, race/ethnicity, and socioeconomic position. Sleep Medicine, 18, 7–18. https://doi.org/10.1016/j.sleep.2015.01.020. Epub 2015 February 28. PMID: 26431755; PMCID: PMC4631795.

Grant, S. F., Li, M., Bradfield, J. P., Kim, C. E., Annaiah, K., Santa, E., Glessner, J. T., Casalunovo, T., Frackelton, E. C., Otieno, F. G., Shaner, J. L., Smith, R. M., Imielinski M, Eckert, A. W., Chiavacci, R. M., Berkowitz, R. I., & Hakonarson, H. (2008, March 12). Association analysis of the FTO gene with obesity in children of Caucasian and African ancestry reveals a common tagging SNP. PLoS One, 3(3), e1746. https://doi.org/10.1371/journal.pone.0001746. PMID: 18335027; PMCID: PMC2262153.

Gruber, K. J., & Haldeman, L. A. (2009). Using the family to combat childhood and adult obesity. Preventing Chronic Disease, 6(3), A106. http://www.cdc.gov/pcd/issues/2009/.

Gu, F., Han, J., Laden, F., Pan, A., Caporaso, N. E., Stampfer, M. J., Kawachi, I., Rexrode, K. M., Willett, W. C., Hankinson, S. E., Speizer, F. E., & Schernhammer, E. S. (2015, March). Total and cause-specific mortality of U.S. nurses working rotating night shifts. American Journal of Preventive Medicine, 48(3), 241–252. https://doi.org/10.1016/j.amepre.2014.10.018. Epub 2015 January 6. PMID: 25576495; PMCID: PMC4339532.

Hahn, R. A. (2021). What is a social determinant of health? Back to basics. Journal of Public Health Research, 10(4), 2324. https://doi.org/10.4081/jphr.2021.2324. PMID: 34162174; PMCID: PMC8672311.

Haleem, A., Javaid, M., Singh, R. P., & Suman, R. (2021). Telemedicine for healthcare: Capabilities, features, barriers, and applications. Sensors International, 2, 100117. https://doi.org/10.1016/j.sintl.2021.100117.

Hales, C. M., Gu, Q., Ogden, C. L., & Yanovski, S. Z. (2022). Use of prescription medications associated with weight gain among US adults, 1999–2018: A nationally representative survey. Obesity, 30(1), 229–239.

Halilagic, A., & Moschonis, G. (2021, September 29). The effect of growth rate during infancy on the risk of developing obesity in childhood: A systematic literature review. Nutrients, 13(10), 3449. https://doi.org/10.3390/nu13103449. PMID: 34684450; PMCID: PMC8537274.

Hall, K. D., & Guo, J. (2017, May). Obesity energetics: Body weight regulation and the effects of diet composition. Gastroenterology, 152(7), 1718–1727.e3. https://doi.org/10.1053/j.gastro.2017.01.052. Epub 2017 February 11. PMID: 28193517; PMCID: PMC5568065.

Hall, R. R., Francis, S., Whitt-Glover, M., Loftin-Bell, K., Swett, K., & McMichael, A. J. (2013). Hair care practices as a barrier to physical activity in African American women. JAMA Dermatology, 149(3), 310–314. https://doi.org/10.1001/jamadermatol.2013.194.

Hall, W. J., Chapman, M. V., Lee, K. M., et al. (2015). Implicit racial/ethnic bias among healthcare professionals and its influence on health care outcomes: A systematic review. American Journal of Public Health, 105(12), e60–e76. https://doi.org/10.2105/AJPH.2015.302903.

Hamman, R. F., Bell, R. A., Dabelea, D., et al. (2014). The SEARCH for diabetes in youth study: Rationale, findings, and future directions. Diabetes Care, 37(12), 3336–3344. https://doi.org/10.2337/dc14-0574. PMID: 25414389; PMCID: PMC4237981.

Hamzeh, N., Ghadimi, F., Farzaneh, R., & Hosseini, S. K. (2017). Obesity, heart failure, and obesity paradox. Journal of Tehran Heart Center, 12(1), 1–5. https://doi.org/10.18502/jthc.v12i1.688.

Hargreaves, M. K., et al. (2020). Cultural tailoring and community engagement: Effective strategies for behavioral interventions in the Black community. Journal of Behavioral Health Services & Research, 47(4), 619–632.

Hart, C. N., Carskadon, M. A., Considine, R. V., Fava, J. L., Lawton, J., Raynor, H. A., Jelalian, E., Owens, J., & Wing, R. (2013, December). Changes in children's sleep duration on food intake, weight, and leptin. Pediatrics, 132(6), e1473–e1480. https://doi.org/10.1542/peds.2013-1274. Epub 2013 November 4. PMID: 24190680.

Hebebrand, J., Friedel, S., Schäuble, N., Geller, F., & Hinney, A. (2003, August). Perspectives: Molecular genetic research in human obesity. Obesity Reviews, 4(3), 139–146. https://doi.org/10.1046/j.1467-789x.2003.00106.x. PMID: 12916815.

Heianza, Y., & Qi, L. (2017). Gene-diet interaction and precision nutrition in obesity. International Journal of Molecular Sciences, 18(4), 787. https://doi.org/10.3390/ijms18040787. PMID: 28387720; PMCID: PMC5412371.

Hernandez, D. C., Reesor, L. M., & Murillo, R. (2017). Food insecurity and adult overweight/obesity: Gender and race/ethnic disparities. Appetite, 117, 373–378. https://doi.org/10.1016/j.appet.2017.07.010.

Hernandez, W., Gamazon, E. R., Smithberger, E., O'Brien, T. J., Harralson, A. F., Tuck, M., Barbour, A., Kittles, R. A., Cavallari, L. H., & Perera, M. A. (2016, April 14). Novel genetic predictors of venous thromboembolism risk in African Americans. Blood, 127(15), 1923–1929. https://doi.org/10.1182/blood-2015-09-668525. Epub 2016 February 17. PMID: 26888256; PMCID: PMC4832509.

Hickson, J., et al. (2024). Navigating the complexity of applying nutrition evidence to practice: A position paper of the Academy of Nutrition and Dietetics. Journal of the Academy of Nutrition and Dietetics, 124(2), 1–10.

Holt, C. L., Clark, E. M., & Roth, D. L. (2014). Positive and negative religious coping and well-being in African Americans: Modeling resources and stressors in a national sample. Journal for the Scientific Study of Religion, 53(3), 539–557. https://doi.org/10.1111/jssr.12145.

Isganaitis, E., Suehiro, H., & Cardona, C. (2017, February). Who's your daddy? Paternal inheritance of metabolic disease risk. Current Opinion in Endocrinology, Diabetes and Obesity, 24(1), 47–55. https://doi.org/10.1097/MED.0000000000000307. PMID: 27906710.

Ivezaj, V., Lydecker, J. A., & Grilo, C. M. (2020, August). Language matters: Patients' preferred terms for discussing obesity and disordered eating with health care providers after bariatric surgery. Obesity (Silver Spring), 28(8), 1412–1418. https://doi.org/10.1002/oby.22868. Epub 2020 July 13. PMID: 32662251; PMCID: PMC7501175.

Jaffee, S. R., & Christian, C. W. (2019). The biological embedding of child abuse and neglect: Implications for policy and practice. Social Policy Report, 32(1), 1–36. https://doi.org/10.1002/sop2.2.

James, D. C. S., Harville, C., Efunbumi, O., & Martin, M. Y. (2015). Health literacy issues surrounding weight management among African American women: A mixed methods study. Journal of Human Nutrition and Dietetics, 28(s2), 41–49. https://doi.org/10.1111/jhn.12239.

Jensen, S. B. K., et al. (2024). Healthy weight loss maintenance with exercise, GLP-1 receptor agonist, or both combined followed by one year without treatment: A post-treatment analysis of a randomised placebo-controlled trial. eClinicalMedicine, 69, 102475.

Johnson, D. A., Jackson, C. L., Williams, N. J., & Alcántara, C. (2019, July 23). Are sleep patterns influenced by race/ethnicity—A marker of relative advantage or disadvantage? Evidence to date. Nature and Science of Sleep, 11, 79–95. https://doi.org/10.2147/NSS.S169312. PMID: 31440109; PMCID: PMC6664254.

Johnson, S., Hill, R., Cook, T., & Hobson, L. (2024). Comment on: Beyond race: social vulnerability and access to metabolic and bariatric surgery. Surgery for Obesity and Related Diseases, 20(12), e23–e24.

Johnson, V. R., Washington, T. B., Chhabria, S., Wang, E. H., Czepiel, K., Reyes, K. J. C., & Stanford, F. C. (2022, May). Food as medicine for obesity treatment and management. Clinical Therapeutics, 44(5), 671–681. https://doi.org/10.1016/j.clinthera.2022.05.001. Epub 2022 May 23. PMID: 35618570; PMCID: PMC9908371.

Johnston, B. C., Kanters, S., Bandayrel, K., et al. (2014). Comparison of weight loss among named diet programs in overweight and obese adults: A meta-analysis. JAMA, 312(9), 923–933. https://doi.org/10.1001/jama.2014.10397.

Joo, J. Y., & Liu, M. F. (2021, September). Culturally tailored interventions for ethnic minorities: A scoping review. Nursing Open, 8(5), 2078–2090. https://doi.org/10.1002/nop2.733. Epub 2020 December 9. PMID: 34388862; PMCID: PMC8363345.

Joseph, R. P., Ainsworth, B. E., Keller, C., & Dodgson, J. E. (2015). Barriers to physical activity among African American women: An integrative review of the literature. Women Health, 55(6), 679–699. https://doi.org/10.1080/03630242.2015.1039184. Epub 2015 April 24. PMID: 25909603; PMCID: PMC4516615.

Kabakambira, J. D., Baker, R. L. Jr, Briker, S. M., et al. (2018). Do current guidelines for waist circumference apply to Black Africans? Prediction of insulin resistance by waist circumference among Africans living in America. BMJ Global Health, 3(5), e001057. https://doi.org/10.1136/bmjgh-2018-001057.

Katzmarzyk, P. T., Martin, C. K., Newton, R. L. Jr, et al. (2018). Promoting successful weight loss in primary care in Louisiana (PROPEL): Rationale, design, and baseline characteristics. Contemporary Clinical Trials, 67, 1–10. https://doi.org/10.1016/j.cct.2018.02.002.

Kaur, Y., De Souza, R. J., Gibson, W. T., & Meyre, D. (2017). A systematic review of genetic syndromes with obesity. Obesity Reviews, 18(6), 603–634.

Kiefner-Burmeister, A., & Hinman, N. (2020, March). The role of general parenting style in child diet and obesity risk. Current Nutrition Reports, 9(1), 14–30. https://doi.org/10.1007/s13668-020-00301-9. PMID: 31960342.

Kitzman, H., et al. (2021). Better me within randomized trial: Faith-based diabetes prevention program for weight loss in African American women. American Journal of Health Promotion, 35(2), 202–213.

Kobylińska, M., Antosik, K., Decyk, A., Kurowska, K. (2022). Malnutrition in obesity: Is it possible? Obes Facts, 15(1), 19–25. https://doi.org/10.1159/000519503. Epub 2021 November 8. PMID: 34749356; PMCID: PMC8820192.

Koyanagi, A., Smith, L., Oh, H., Yang, L., Jackson, S. E., Haro, J. M., Shin, J. I. I., Carvalho, A. F., & Jacob, L. (2020, October 29). Secondhand smoking and obesity among nonsmoking adolescents aged 12–15 years from 38 low- and middle-income countries. Nicotine & Tobacco Research, 22(11), 2014–2021. https://doi.org/10.1093/ntr/ntaa053. PMID: 32211794; PMCID: PMC7593363.

Krist, A. H., Tong, S. T., Aycock, R. A., & Longo, D. R. (2017). Engaging patients in decision-making and behavior change to promote prevention. Studies in Health Technology and Informatics, 240, 284–302. PMID: 28972524; PMCID: PMC6996004.

Krueger, P. M., & Reither, E. N. (2015, November). Mind the gap: Race/ethnic and socioeconomic disparities in obesity. Current Diabetes Reports, 15(11), 95. https://doi.org/10.1007/s11892-015-0666-6. PMID: 26377742; PMCID: PMC4947380.

Kumar, S., & Kelly, A. S. (2017, February). Review of childhood obesity: From epidemiology, etiology, and comorbidities to clinical assessment and treatment. In Mayo Clinic Proceedings (Vol. 92, No. 2, pp. 251–265). Elsevier.

Kuna, S. T., Reboussin, D. M., Borradaile, K. E., et al. (2013). Long-term effect of weight loss on obstructive sleep apnea severity in obese patients with type 2 diabetes. Sleep, 36, 641.

Kühnen, P., Biebermann, H., & Wiegand, S. (2022). Pharmacotherapy in childhood obesity. Hormone Research in Paediatrics, 95(2), 177–192.

Latomme, J., Morgan, P. J., Chastin, S., Brondeel, R., & Cardon, G. (2023, February 15). Effects of a family-based lifestyle intervention on co-physical activity and other health-related outcomes of fathers and their children: The 'Run Daddy Run' intervention. BMC Public Health, 23(1), 342. https://doi.org/10.1186/s12889-023-15191-z. PMID: 36793044; PMCID: PMC9930712.

Lawlor, D., Relton, C., Sattar, N., et al. (2012). Maternal adiposity—A determinant of perinatal and offspring outcomes? Nature Reviews Endocrinology, 8, 679–688. https://doi.org/10.1038/nrendo.2012.176.

Lee, A., Cardel, M., & Donahoo, W. T. (2019, October 12). Social and environmental factors influencing obesity. In Feingold, K. R., Anawalt, B., Blackman, M. R., et al., editors. Endotext [Internet]. South Dartmouth, MA: MDText.com, Inc; 2000. https://www.ncbi.nlm.nih.gov/books/NBK278977/.

Leutner, M., Dervic, E., Bellach, L. et al. (2023). Obesity as pleiotropic risk state for metabolic and mental health throughout life. Translational Psychiatry, 13, 175. https://doi.org/10.1038/s41398-023-02447-w.

Lewis, C., Cohen, P. R., Bahl, D., Levine, E. M., & Khaliq, W. (2023, July 1). Race and ethnic categories: A brief review of global terms and nomenclature. Cureus, 15(7), e41253. https://doi.org/10.7759/cureus.41253. PMID: 37529803; PMCID: PMC10389293.

Lewis, K. H., Gudzune, K. A., Fischer, H., Yamamoto, A., & Young, D. R. (2016, June 30). Racial and ethnic minority patients report different weight-related care experiences than non-Hispanic Whites. Preventive Medicine Reports, 4, 296–302. https://doi.org/10.1016/j.pmedr.2016.06.015. PMID: 27486558; PMCID: PMC4960010.

Lianov, L. (2023, June 17). The role of positive psychology in lifestyle medicine. American Journal of Lifestyle Medicine, 18(5), 666–670. https://doi.org/10.1177/15598276231184157. PMID: 39309325; PMCID: PMC11412374.

Lima, R. A., Desoye, G., Simmons, D., et al. (2021). The importance of maternal insulin resistance throughout pregnancy on neonatal adiposity. Paediatric and Perinatal Epidemiology, 35, 83–91. https://doi.org/10.1111/ppe.12682.

Lindberg, L., Hagman, E., Danielsson, P., Marcus, C., & Persson, M. (2020). Anxiety and depression in children and adolescents with obesity: A nationwide study in Sweden. BMC Medicine, 18(1). https://doi.org/10.1186/s12916-020-1498-z.

Lindström, M., Rosvall, M., & Pirouzifard, M. (2023). Leisure-time physical activity, desire to increase physical activity, and mortality: A population-based prospective cohort study. Preventive Medicine Reports, 33, 102212. https://doi.org/10.1016/j.pmedr.2023.102212.

Liu, Q., Shi, J., Duan, P., Liu, B., Li, T., Wang, C., Li, H., Yang, T., Gan, Y., Wang, X., Cao, S., & Lu, Z. (2018, December 1). Is shift work associated with a higher risk of overweight or obesity? A systematic review of observational studies with meta-analysis. International Journal of Epidemiology, 47(6), 1956–1971. https://doi.org/10.1093/ije/dyy079. PMID: 29850840.

Lofton, H., Ard, J. D., Hunt, R. R., & Knight, M. G. (2023). Obesity among African American people in the United States: A review. Obesity (Silver Spring), 31(2), 306–315. https://doi.org/10.1002/oby.23640. PMID: 36695059; PMCID: PMC10107750.

Look AHEAD Research Group, Pi-Sunyer, X., Blackburn, G., et al. (2007). Reduction in weight and cardiovascular disease risk factors in individuals with type 2 diabetes: One-year results of the Look AHEAD trial. Diabetes Care, 30, 1374.

Look AHEAD Research Group, Wing, R. R., Bolin, P., et al. (2013). Cardiovascular effects of intensive lifestyle intervention in type 2 diabetes. New England Journal of Medicine, 369, 145.

Lovasi, G. S., Hutson, M. A., Guerra, M., & Neckerman, K. M. (2009, November 1). Built environments and obesity in disadvantaged populations. Epidemiologic Reviews, 31(1), 7–20. https://doi.org/10.1093/epirev/mxp005. Epub 2009 July 9. PMID: 19589839.

Mahmood, L., Flores-Barrantes, P., Moreno, L. A., Manios, Y., & Gonzalez-Gil, E. M. (2021). The influence of parental dietary behaviors and practices on children's eating habits. Nutrients, 13(4), 1138.

Mahmood, S., Li, Y., & Hynes, M. (2023). Adverse childhood experiences and obesity: A one-to-one correlation? Clinical Child Psychology and Psychiatry, 28(2), 785–794. https://doi.org/10.1177/13591045221119001.

Mahmoud, A. M. (2022, January 25). An overview of epigenetics in obesity: The role of lifestyle and therapeutic interventions. International Journal of Molecular Sciences, 23(3), 1341. https://doi.org/10.3390/ijms23031341. PMID: 35163268; PMCID: PMC8836029.

Mallik, R., Carpenter, J., & Zalin, A. (2023, July). Assessment of obesity. Clinical Medicine (London), 23(4), 299–303. https://doi.org/10.7861/clinmed.2023-0148. PMID: 37524433; PMCID: PMC10541030.

Mandy, M., & Nyirenda, M. (2018). Developmental origins of health and disease: The relevance to developing nations. International Health, 10, 66–70.

Mantena, S., & Keshavjee, S. (2021, July). Strengthening healthcare delivery with remote patient monitoring in the time of COVID-19. BMJ Health & Care Informatics, 28, e100302. https://doi.org/10.1136/bmjhci-2021-100302. PMID: 34289962; PMCID: PMC8300556.

Martínez-González, M. A., Gea, A., & Ruiz-Canela, M. (2019). The Mediterranean diet and cardiovascular health. Circulation Research, 124(5), 779–798. https://doi.org/10.1161/CIRCRESAHA.118.313348. PMID: 30817261.

Mattingly, T. J., Hyman, D. A., & Bai, G. (2023). Pharmacy benefit managers: History, business practices, economics, and policy. JAMA Health Forum, 4(11), e233804. https://doi.org/10.1001/jamahealthforum.2023.3804.

McIntyre, R. S., Kwan, A. T. H., Rosenblat, J. D., Teopiz, K. M., & Mansur, R. B. (2024, January 1). Psychotropic drug-related weight gain and its treatment. American Journal of Psychiatry, 181(1), 26–38. https://doi.org/10.1176/appi.ajp.20230922. PMID: 38161305.

Mechanick, J. I., Butsch, W. S., Christensen, S. M., Hamdy, O., Li, Z., Prado, C. M., & Heymsfield, S. B. (2024, September 19). Strategies for minimizing muscle loss during use of incretin-mimetic drugs for treatment of obesity. Obesity Reviews, e13841. https://doi.org/10.1111/obr.13841. Epub ahead of print. PMID: 39295512.

Melamed, O. C., Selby, P., & Taylor, V. H. (2022). Mental health and obesity during the COVID-19 pandemic. Current Obesity Reports, 11, 23–31. https://doi.org/10.1007/s13679-021-00466-6.

Mensinger, J. L., Tylka, T. L., & Calamari, M. E. (2018, June). Mechanisms underlying weight status and healthcare avoidance in women: A study of weight stigma, body-related shame and guilt, and healthcare stress. Body Image, 25, 139–147. https://doi.org/10.1016/j.bodyim.2018.03.001. Epub 2018 Mar 22. PMID: 29574257.

Mikulska, J., Juszczyk, G., Gawrońska-Grzywacz, M., & Herbet, M. (2021, September 30). HPA axis in the pathomechanism of depression and schizophrenia: New therapeutic strategies based on its participation. Brain Sciences, 11(10), 1298. https://doi.org/10.3390/brainsci11101298. PMID: 34679364; PMCID: PMC8533829.

Miller, A. L., Lumeng, J. C., & LeBourgeois, M. K. (2015, February). Sleep patterns and obesity in childhood. Current Opinion in Endocrinology, Diabetes and Obesity, 22(1), 41–47. https://doi.org/10.1097/MED.0000000000000125. PMID: 25517022; PMCID: PMC4437224.

Miller, W. R. (2023). The evolution of motivational interviewing. Behavioural and Cognitive Psychotherapy, 51(6), 616–632. https://doi.org/10.1017/S1352465822000431.

Miller, W. R., & Rollnick, S. (2021). Motivational interviewing: Helping people change (3rd ed.). Guilford Press.

Minihan, P. M., Fitch, S. N., & Must, A. (2007). What does the epidemic of childhood obesity mean for children with special health care needs? Journal of Law, Medicine & Ethics, 35(1), 61–77. https://doi.org/10.1111/j.1748-720X.2007.00113.x.

Mohammadian Khonsari, N., Shahrestanaki, E., Ehsani, A., Asadi, S., Sokoty, L., Mohammadpoor Nami, S., Hakak-Zargar, B., & Qorbani, M. (2023). Association of childhood and adolescence obesity with incidence and mortality of adulthood cancers. A systematic review and meta-analysis. Frontiers in Endocrinology, 14, 1069164. https://doi.org/10.3389/fendo.2023.1069164. PMID: 36742402; PMCID: PMC9892178.

Mohammed, S. H., Habtewold, T. D., Birhanu, M. M., Sissay, T. A., Tegegne, B. S., Abuzerr, S., & Esmaillzadeh, A. (2019). Neighbourhood socioeconomic status and overweight/obesity: A systematic review and meta-analysis of epidemiological studies. BMJ Open, 9(11), e028238. https://doi.org/10.1136/bmjopen-2018-028238. PMID: 31727643; PMCID: PMC6886990.

Möller, F., Hedberg, J., Skogar, M., & Sundbom, M. (2023, October). Long-term follow-up 15 years after duodenal switch or gastric bypass for super obesity: A randomized controlled trial. Obesity Surgery, 33(10), 2981–2990. https://doi.org/10.1007/s11695-023-06767-0. Epub 2023 August 16. PMID: 37584851; PMCID: PMC10514119.

Mourino, N., Pérez-Ríos, M., Yolton, K., Lanphear, B. P., Chen, A., Buckley, J. P., Kalkwarf, H. J., Cecil, K. M., & Braun, J. M. (2022 August). Pre- and postnatal exposure to secondhand tobacco smoke and body composition at 12 years: Periods of susceptibility. Obesity (Silver Spring), 30(8), 1659–1669. https://doi.org/10.1002/oby.23480. PMID: 35894081; PMCID: PMC9335905.

Mulholland, R. S., Paul, M. D., & Chalfoun, C. (2016). Noninvasive body contouring with radiofrequency, ultrasound, cryolipolysis, and low-level laser therapy. Clinics in Plastic Surgery, 43(4), 643–654.

Muscat, D. M., Shepherd, H. L., Nutbeam, D., Trevena, L., & McCaffery, K. J. (2021). Health literacy and shared decision-making: Exploring the relationship to enable meaningful patient engagement in healthcare. Journal of General Internal Medicine, 36, 521–524.

Music Milanovic, S., Buoncristiano, M., Krizan, H., Rathmes, G., & Williams, C. (2021). Socioeconomic disparities in physical activity, sedentary behavior, and sleep patterns among 6–9 year old children from 24 countries in the WHO European region. Obesiy Reviews, 22(Suppl 6), e13209

Must, A., Phillips, S. M., & Naumova, E. N. (2012). Occurrence and timing of childhood overweight and mortality: Findings from the Third Harvard Growth Study. Journal of Pediatrics, 160(5), 743–750. https://doi.org/10.1016/j.jpeds.2011.10.037.

Muth, N. D., Dietz, W. H., Magge, S. N., & Johnson, R. K. (2019, April). Public policies to reduce sugary drink consumption in children and adolescents. Pediatrics, 143(4), e20190282.

National Academies of Sciences, Engineering, and Medicine; Health and Medicine Division; Board on Population Health and Public Health Practice; Committee on Community-Based Solutions to Promote Health Equity in the United States; Baciu, A., Negussie, Y., Geller, A., et al., editors. (2017). Communities in action: Pathways to health equity. Washington, DC: National Academies Press (US). https://www.ncbi.nlm.nih.gov/books/NBK425849/.

National Association to Advance Fat Acceptance (NAAFA). (2024). NAAFA. https://naafa.org/.

Nduma, B. N., Mofor, K. A., Tatang, J., Amougou, L., Nkeonye, S., Chineme, P., Ekhator, C., & Ambe, S. (2023, July 6). Endoscopic sleeve gastroplasty (ESG) vesus laparoscopic sleeve gastroplasty (LSG): A comparative review. Cureus, 15(7), e41466. https://doi.org/10.7759/cureus.41466. PMID: 37426405; PMCID: PMC10325692.

Nogueira, M., Teixeira, D., Pires, B., Mosca, S., Teixeira, A. L., Clemente, F., & Sevivas, F. (2023). Mental health and coping strategies used by nurses during the COVID-19 pandemic: Scoping review. Journal of Social and Educational Research, 2(1), 1–7.

Noonan, A. S., Velasco-Mondragon, H. E., & Wagner, F. A. (2016, October 3). Improving the health of African Americans in the USA: An overdue opportunity for social justice. Public Health Reviews, 37, 12. https://doi.org/10.1186/s40985-016-0025-4. PMID: 29450054; PMCID: PMC5810013.

O'Connor, T. G. (2017). Updating biological bases of social behavior. Journal of Child Psychology and Psychiatry, 55, 957–958. https://doi.org/10.1111/jcpp.12313.

OAC Online Survey. (2020). OAC online survey of 1,114 U.S. adults, May 2020; OAC online survey of 517 U.S. Black/African American adults, August 2020; OAC online survey of 530 U.S. Latino/Hispanic adults, August 2020; OAC online survey of 429 U.S. Asian/Pacific Islander adults, August 2020.

Obesity Medicine Association. (2022). Obesity consensus statement. Obesity Medicine Association. Retrieved October 28, 2024, from https://obesitymedicine. org/about/obesity-consensus-statement/

Obita, G., & Alkhatib, A. (2022, July 6). Disparities in the prevalence of childhood obesity-related comorbidities: A systematic review. Frontiers in Public Health, 10, 923744. https://doi.org/10.3389/fpubh.2022.923744. PMID: 35874993; PMCID: PMC9298527.

Ogden, C. L., Fryar, C. D., Hales, C. M., Carroll, M. D., Aoki, Y., & Freedman, D. S. (2018). Differences in obesity prevalence by demographics and urbanization in US children and adolescents, 2013–2016. JAMA, 319(23), 2410–2418. https:// doi.org/10.1001/jama.2018.5158.

Okobi, O. E., Beeko, P. K. A., Nikravesh, E., Beeko, M. A. E., Ofiaeli, C., Ojinna, B. T., Okunromade, O., Dick, A. I., Sulaiman, A. R., & Sowemimo, A. (2023). Trends in obesity-related mortality and racial disparities. Cureus, 15(7), e41432. https://doi.org/10.7759/cureus.41432.

Omoisilli, O. E., Goodman, A. B., Dooyema, C. A., Harrison, M. R., Belay, B., & Park, S. (2019, February). Screening and referral for childhood obesity: Adherence to the U.S. Preventive Services Task Force recommendation. American Journal of Preventive Medicine, 56(2), 179–186. https://doi.org/10.1016/j.amepre.2018. 10.003. Epub 2018 Dec 17. PMID: 30573333; PMCID: PMC10863670.

Papatriantafyllou, E., Efthymiou, D., Zoumbaneas, E., Popescu, C. A., & Vassilopoulou, E. (2022, April 8). Sleep deprivation: Effects on weight loss and weight loss maintenance. Nutrients, 14(8), 1549. https://doi.org/10.3390/nu14081549. PMID: 35458110; PMCID: PMC9031614.

Paradies, Y. (2015, September 23). Racism as a determinant of health: A systematic review and meta-analysis. PLoS One, 10(9), e0138511. https://doi.org/10.1371/ journal.pone.0138511. PMID: 26398658; PMCID: PMC4580597.

Pati, S., Irfan, W., Jameel, A., Ahmed, S., & Shahid, R. K. (2023). Obesity and cancer: A current overview of epidemiology, pathogenesis, outcomes, and management. Cancers, 15(2), 485. https://doi.org/10.3390/cancers15020485.

Pearl, R. L., & Puhl, R. M. (2018). Weight bias internalization and health: A systematic review. Obesity Reviews, 19(8), 1141–1163. https://doi.org/10.1111/obr.12701.

Phelan, S. M., Burgess, D. J., Yeazel, M. W., Hellerstedt, W. L., Griffin, J. M., & van Ryn, M. (2015, April). Impact of weight bias and stigma on quality of care and outcomes for patients with obesity. Obesity Reviews, 16(4), 319–326. https:// doi.org/10.1111/obr.12266. Epub 2015 March 5. PMID: 25752756; PMCID: PMC4381543.

Post, R. E., Mainous, A. G. III, Gregorie, S. H., Knoll, M. E., Diaz, V. A., & Saxena, S. K. (2011). The influence of physician acknowledgment of patients' weight status on patient perceptions of overweight and obesity in the United States. Archives of Internal Medicine, 171, 316–321.

Preventive care and screening: Body mass index (BMI) screening and follow-up plan. (n.d.). Retrieved January 26, 2023, from https://qpp.cms.gov/docs/ecqm-specs/2017/EC_CMS69v5_NQF0421_BMI_and_Follow_Up/CMS69v5.html.

Prochaska, J. O., & DiClemente, C. C. (1983). Stages and processes of self-change of smoking: Toward an integrative model of change. Journal of Consulting and Clinical Psychology, 51(3), 390–395.

Pronk, N., Kleinman, D. V., Goekler, S. F., Ochiai, E., Blakey, C., Brewer, K. H. (2021). Promoting health and well-being in healthy people 2030. Journal of Public Health Management and Practice, 27(Supplement 6), S242–S248. https://doi.org/10.1097/PHH.0000000000001254.

Puhl, R. M., Lessard, L. M., Himmelstein, M. S., & Foster, G. D. (2021, June 1). The roles of experienced and internalized weight stigma in healthcare experiences: Perspectives of adults engaged in weight management across six countries. PLoS One, 16(6), e0251566. https://doi.org/10.1371/journal.pone.0251566. PMID: 34061867; PMCID: PMC8168902.

Puhl, R. M., & Heuer, C. A. (2010). Obesity stigma: Important considerations for public health. American Journal of Public Health, 100(6), 1019–1028. https://doi.org/10.2105/AJPH.2009.159491. Epub 2010 January 14. PMID: 20075322; PMCID: PMC2866597.

Puhl, R. M., Phelan, S. M., Nadglowski, J., & Kyle, T. K. (2016). Overcoming weight bias in the management of patients with diabetes and obesity. Clinical Diabetes, 34(1), 44–50. https://doi.org/10.2337/diaclin.34.1.44.

Randal, C., Pratt, D., & Bucci, S. (2015). Mindfulness and self-esteem: A systematic review. Mindfulness, 6, 1366–1378. https://doi.org/10.1007/s12671-015-0407-6.

Rettner, R. (2012). Hair concerns keep some woman for gym. NBC News. https://.www.nbcnews.com/health/health-news/hair-issues-make-some-black-women-exercise-less-flna1c7663596.

Rhemtulla, I. A., Vonderhaar, R. J., Mauch, J. T., Broach, R. B., Familusi, O., & Butler, P. D. (2019). Improvement in racial disparity among patients undergoing panniculectomy after bariatric surgery. American Journal of Surgery, 218(1), 37–41. ISSN 0002-9610. https://doi.org/10.1016/j.amjsurg.2019.01.002. https://www.sciencedirect.com/science/article/pii/S0002961018308869.

Rippe, J. M. (2018, December 2). Lifestyle strategies for risk factor reduction, prevention, and treatment of cardiovascular disease. American Journal of Lifestyle Medicine, 13(2), 204–212. https://doi.org/10.1177/1559827618812395. PMID: 30800027; PMCID: PMC6378495.

Riser, T. J., Thompson, R. A., Curtis, C., Squires, A., Mowinski Jennings, B., & Szanton, S. L. (2023). Freedom is not free: Examining health equity for racial and ethnic minoritized veterans. Research in Nursing & Health, 46(2), 181–185. https://doi.org/10.1002/nur.22304.

Robinson, T. N., Callister, R., & Berry, D. C. (2020). The role of media in shaping perceptions of race and obesity: The case of "body positivity." Journal of Health Communication, 25(3), 198–206. https://doi.org/10.1080/10810730.2020.1752485.

Rojo, M., Solano, S., Lacruz, T., Baile, J. I., Blanco, M., Graell, M., & Sepúlveda, A. R. (2021, March 10). Linking psychosocial stress events, psychological disorders and childhood obesity. Children (Basel), 8(3), 211. https://doi.org/10.3390/children8030211. PMID: 33802090; PMCID: PMC8000555.

Rotimi, C. N., Tekola-Ayele, F., Baker, J. L., & Shriner, D. (2016, December). The African Diaspora: History, adaptation and health. Current Opinion in Genetics & Development, 41, 77–84. https://doi.org/10.1016/j.gde.2016.08.005. Epub 2016 September 16. PMID: 27644073; PMCID: PMC5318189.

Ruan, X., Li, R., Wang, L., Lu, S., Wen, A., Sameer, M., & Liu, H. (2024). Current status of anti-obesity medications and performance, an EHR-based survey. medRxiv, 2024-12.

Rubak, S., Sandbaek, A., Lauritzen, T., & Christensen, B. (2005). Motivational interviewing: A systematic review and meta-analysis. British Journal of General Practice, 55(513), 305–312.

Rubino, D., Neff, K. J., Haqq, A. M., Ryder, J. R., Kelly, A. S., Pietrobelli, A., . . . Yanovski, J. A. (2023). Tirzepatide for the treatment of obesity in adolescents. New England Journal of Medicine, 389(15), 1393–1404. https://doi.org/10.1056/NEJMoa2307563.

Sadeghi, H. M., Adeli, I., Calina, D., Docea, A. O., Mousavi, T., Daniali, M., Nikfar, S., Tsatsakis, A., & Abdollahi, M. (2022). Polycystic ovary syndrome: A comprehensive review of pathogenesis, management, and drug repurposing. International Journal of Molecular Sciences, 23(2), 583. https://doi.org/10.3390/ijms23020583.

Sadeghi, P., Duarte-Bateman, D., Ma, W., Khalaf, R., Fodor, R., Pieretti, G., Ciccarelli, F., Harandi, H., & Cuomo, R. (2022). Post-bariatric plastic surgery: Abdominoplasty, the state of the art in body contouring. Journal of Clinical Medicine, 11(15), 4315. https://doi.org/10.3390/jcm11154315.

Sadeghi, S., Pouretemad, H., Khosrowabadi, R., Fathabadi, J., & Nikbakht, S. (2019, October). Behavioral and electrophysiological evidence for parent training in young children with autism symptoms and excessive screen-time. Asian Journal of Psychiatry, 45, 7–12. https://doi.org/10.1016/j.ajp.2019.08.003. Epub 2019 August 5. PMID: 31430692.

Sarna, S. K., & Otterson, M. F. (1989). Small intestinal physiology and pathophysiology. Gastroenterology Clinics of North America, 18(2), 375–404. https://doi.org/10.1016/S0889-8553(21)00452-6.

Sart, G., Bayar, Y., & Danilina, M. (2023). Impact of educational attainment and economic globalization on obesity in adult females and males: Empirical evidence from BRICS economies. Frontiers in Public Health, 11, 1102359.

Saulle, R., Bernardi, M., Chiarini, M., Backhaus, I., & La Torre, G. (2018). Shift work, overweight and obesity in health professionals: A systematic review and meta-analysis. Clinical Therapeutics, 169(4), e189–e197. https://doi.org/10.7417/T.2018.2077. PMID: 30151553.

Saunders, K. H., et al. (2016). Drug-induced weight gain: Rethinking our choices. Journal of Family Practice, 65(11), 780–788.

Shai, I., Schwarzfuchs, D., Henkin, Y., et al. (2008). Weight loss with a low-carbohydrate, Mediterranean, or low-fat diet. New England Journal of Medicine, 359, 229.

Shakya, A., Goren, A., Shalek, A., German, C. N., Snook, J., Kuchroo, V. K., Yosef, N., Chan, R. C., Regev, A., Williams, M. A., & Tantin, D. (2015, November 16). Oct1 and OCA-B are selectively required for CD4 memory T cell function. Journal of Experimental Medicine, 212(12), 2115–2131. https://doi.org/10.1084/jem.20150363. Epub 2015 October 19. PMID: 26481684; PMCID: PMC4647264.

Shan, Z., Guo, Y., Hu, F. B., Liu, L., & Qi, Q. (2020). Association of low-carbohydrate and low-fat diets with mortality among US adults. JAMA Internal Medicine, 180(4), 513–523. https://doi.org/10.1001/jamainternmed.2019.6980. PMID: 31961383; PMCID: PMC6990856.

Shrivastava, A., & Johnston, M. E. (2010, January). Weight-gain in psychiatric treatment: Risks, implications, and strategies for prevention and management. Mens Sana Monographs, 8(1), 53–68. https://doi.org/10.4103/0973-1229.58819. PMID: 21327170; PMCID: PMC3031940.

Smith, J. D., Fu, E., & Kobayashi, M. A. (2020). Prevention and management of childhood obesity and its psychological and health comorbidities. Annual Review of Clinical Psychology, 16(1), 351–378.

Spinner J. R. (2022). An examination of the impact of social and cultural traditions contributing to overweight and obesity among black women. Journal of Primary Care and Community Health. 13. doi.10.1177/21501319221098519.

Stanford, F. C., Lee, M., & Hur, C. (2019). Race, ethnicity, sex, and obesity: Is it time to personalize the scale? Mayo Clinic Proceedings, 94(2), 362–363. Doi: 10.1016/j.mayocp.2018.10.014. PMID: PMC6818706.

Strings, S. (2019a). Fearing the Black body: The racial origins of fat phobia. NYU Press.

Strings, S. (2019b, July 6). The racist roots of fighting obesity. Scientific American. https://www.scientificamerican.com/article/the-racist-roots-of-fighting-obesity2/.

Strings, S. (2020, September). Fearing the Black body: The racial origins of fat phobia. Social Forces, 99(1), e3. https://doi.org/10.1093/sf/soz161.

Sturm, R., & An, R. (2014, September–October). Obesity and economic environments. CA: A Cancer Journal of Clinician, 64(5), 337–350. https://doi.org/10.3322/caac.21237. Epub 2014 May 22. PMID: 24853237; PMCID: PMC4159423.

Swift, D. L., Johannsen, N. M., Lavie, C. J., Earnest, C. P., & Church, T. S. (2014). The role of exercise and physical activity in weight loss and maintenance. Progress in Cardiovascular Diseases, 56(4), 441–447. https://doi.org/10.1016/j.pcad.2013.09.012.

Tahir, M. J., Willett, W., & Forman, M. R. (2019, February 1). The association of television viewing in childhood with overweight and obesity throughout the life course. American Journal of Epidemiology, 188(2), 282–293. https://doi.org/10.1093/aje/kwy236. PMID: 30321270; PMCID: PMC6357794.

Tate, E. B., Wood, W., Liao, Y., & Dunton, G. F. (2015, May). Do stressed mothers have heavier children? A meta-analysis on the relationship between maternal stress and child body mass index. Obesity Reviews, 16(5), 351–361. https://doi.org/10.1111/obr.12262. PMID: 25879393; PMCID: PMC4447110.

Taveras, E. M., Gillman, M. W., Kleinman, K., Rich-Edwards, J. W., & Rifas-Shiman, S. L. (2010). Racial/ethnic differences in early-life risk factors for childhood obesity. Pediatrics, 125(4), 686–695. https://doi.org/10.1542/peds.2009-2100.

Taveras, E. M., Marshall, R., Kleinman, K. P., et al. (2015). Comparative effectiveness of childhood obesity interventions in pediatric primary care: A cluster-randomized clinical trial. JAMA Pediatrics, 169(6), 535–542. https://doi.org/10.1001/jamapediatrics.2015.0182.

Taylor, D. J., et al. (2024). Beyond the human genome project: The age of complete human genome sequences and pangenome references. Annual Review of Human Genetics, 25.

Thorpe, K., Toles, A., Shah B., Schneider, J., & Bravata, D. M. (2021). Weight loss-associated decreases in medical care expenditures for commercially insured patients with chronic conditions. Journal of Occupational and Environmental Medicine, 63(10), 847–851. https://doi.org/10.1097/JOM.0000000000002296. PMID: 34138824; PMCID: PMC8478295.

Tilman, R. (Producer), & Tillman, G. (Director). (1997). Soul Food [Film]. Fox 2000 Pictures.

Townshend, T., & Lake, A. (2017). Obesogenic environments: Current evidence of the built and food environments. Perspect Public Health, 137(1), 38–44. https://doi.org/10.1177/1757913916679860. PMID: 28449616.

Tran, L. T., Park, S., Kim, S. K. et al. (2022). Hypothalamic control of energy expenditure and thermogenesis. Experimental & Molecular Medicine, 54, 358–369. https://doi.org/10.1038/s12276-022-00741-z.

Tremblay, M. S., Aubert, S., Barnes, J. D., et al. (2017). Sedentary Behavior Research Network (SBRN): Terminology consensus project process and outcome. International Journal of Behavioral Nutrition and Physical Activity, 14(1), 75.

Trent, M., & Gordon, C. M. (2020). Diagnosis and management of polycystic ovary syndrome in adolescents. Pediatrics, 145(Supplement_2), S210–S218. https://doi.org/10.1542/peds.2019-2056J.

U.S. Department of Health and Human Services. (2018). Physical activity guidelines for Americans (2nd ed.). https://health.gov/sites/default/files/2019-09/Physical_Activity_Guidelines_2nd_edition.pdf.

U.S. Preventive Services Task Force. (2018). Obesity in adults: Interventions. https://www.uspreventiveservicestaskforce.org/uspstf/recommendation/obesity-in-adults-interventions.

Ussery, E. N., Fulton, J. E., Galuska, D. A., Katzmarzyk, P. T., & Carlson, S. A. (2018). Joint prevalence of sitting time and leisure-time physical activity among US adults, 2015–2016. JAMA, 320(19), 2036–2038. https://doi.org/10.1001/jama.2018.17797.

Van Dijk, S. J., Tellam, R. L., Morrison, J. L., et al. (2015). Recent developments on the role of epigenetics in obesity and metabolic disease. Clinical Epigenetics, 7, 66. https://doi.org/10.1186/s13148-015-0101-5.

Vedovato, G. M., Surkan, P. J., Jones-Smith, J., Steeves, E. A., Han, E., Trude, A. C., Kharmats, A. Y., & Gittelsohn, J. (2016, June). Food insecurity, overweight and obesity among low-income African-American families in Baltimore City: Associations with food-related perceptions. Public Health Nutrition, 19(8), 1405–1416. https://doi.org/10.1017/S1368980015002888. Epub 2015 October 6. PMID: 26441159; PMCID: PMC4823174.

Vega-Diaz, et al. (2023, December 21). Influence of parental involvement and parenting styles in children's active lifestyle: A systematic review. PeerJ, 11, e1668. doi:10.7717/peerj.16668. PMID: 38144179; PMCID: PMC10749091.

Versey, H. S. (2014). Centering perspectives on Black women, hair politics, and physical activity. American Journal of Public Health, 104(10), 173–178. https://doi.org/10.2105/AJPH.2013.301675.

Wall, L. L. (2006). The medical ethics of Dr J Marion Sims: A fresh look at the historical record. Journal of Medical Ethics, 32(6), 346–350.

Ward, S. H., Gray, A. M., & Paranjape, A. (2009, May). African Americans' perceptions of physician attempts to address obesity in the primary care setting. Journal of General Internal Medicine, 24(5), 579–584. https://doi.org/10.1007/s11606-009-0922-z. Epub 2009 March 10. PMID: 19277791; PMCID: PMC2669857.

Ward, Z. J., Bleich, S. N., Cradock, A. L., Barrett, J. L., Giles, C. M., Flax, C., Long, M. W., & Gortmaker, S. L. (2019). Projected U.S. state-level prevalence of adult obesity and severe obesity. New England Journal of Medicine, 381(25), 2440–2450. https://doi.org/10.1056/NEJMsa1909301. PMID: 31851800.

Washington, T. B., Johnson, V. R., Kendrick, K., Ibrahim, A. A., Tu, L., Sun, K., & Stanford, F. C. (2023). Disparities in access and quality of obesity care. Gastroenterology Clinics of North America, 52(2), 429–441.

Weihe, P., Spielmann, J., Kielstein, H., Henning-Klusmann, J., & Weihrauch-Blüher, S. (2020). Childhood obesity and cancer risk in adulthood. Current Obesity Reports, 9(3), 204–212. https://doi.org/10.1007/s13679-020-00387.

Wiss, D. A., & Brewerton, T. D. (2020, September 1). Adverse childhood experiences and adult obesity: A systematic review of plausible mechanisms and meta-analysis of cross-sectional studies. Physiology & Behavior, 223, 112964. https://doi.org/10.1016/j.physbeh.2020.112964. Epub 2020 May 29. PMID: 32479804.

Wong, M. S., Gudzune, K. A., & Bleich, S. N. (2015, April). Provider communication quality: Influence of patients' weight and race. Patient Education and Counseling, 98(4), 492–498. https://doi.org/10.1016/j.pec.2014.12.007. Epub 2015 January 7. PMID: 25617907; PMCID: PMC4379992.

Wright, D. R., Guo, J., & Hernandez, I. (2023). A prescription for achieving equitable access to anti-obesity medications. JAMA Health Forum, 4(4), e230493. https://doi.org/10.1001/jamahealthforum.2023.0493.

Yancy, G. (2020). Black disciplinary zones and the exposure of whiteness. Educational Philosophy and Theory, 53(3), 217–226. https://doi.org/10.1080/00131857.2020.1830062.

Yancy, W. S., Olsen, M. K., Guyton, J. R., et al. (2004). A low-carbohydrate, ketogenic diet versus a low-fat diet to treat obesity and hyperlipidemia: A randomized, controlled trial. Annals of Internal Medicine, 140, 769–777. https://doi.org/10.7326/0003-4819-140-10-200405180-00006.

Yu, B., Chen, Y., Qin, H., Chen, Q., Wang, J., & Chen, P. (2021, April 15). Using multi-disciplinary teams to treat obese patients helps improve clinical efficacy: The general practitioner's perspective. American Journal of Translational Research, 13(4), 2571–2580. PMID: 34017416; PMCID: PMC8129361.

Yu, Y., Matlin, S. L., Crusto, C. A., Hunter, B., & Tebes, J. K. (2022). Double stigma and help-seeking barriers among Blacks with a behavioral health disorder. Psychiatric Rehabilitation Journal, 45(2), 183–191. https://doi.org/10.1037/prj0000507.

Zajacova, A., & Lawrence, E. M. (2018). The relationship between education and health: Reducing disparities through a contextual approach. Annual Review of Public Health, 39, 273–289. https://doi.org/10.1146/annurev-publhealth-031816-044628. Epub 2018 Jan 12. PMID: 29328865; PMCID: PMC5880718.

Zheng, M., Lamb, K. E., Grimes, C., Laws, R., Bolton, K., Ong, K. K., & Campbell, K. (2018). Rapid weight gain during infancy and subsequent adiposity: A systematic review and meta-analysis of evidence. Obesity Reviews, 19(3), 321–332.

Zielińska, M., Łuszczki, E., Szymańska, A., & Dereń, K. (2024, June 28). Food addiction and the physical and mental health status of adults with overweight and obesity. PeerJ, 12, e17639. https://doi.org/10.7717/peerj.17639. PMID: 38952972; PMCID: PMC11216192.

Index